PELVIC HEALTH
& Childbirth

PELVIC HEALTH
& Childbirth

What Every Woman Needs to Know

MAGNUS MURPHY, M.D.,
and CAROL L. WASSON

Foreword by Linda Brubaker, M.D.,
Female Pelvic Medicine Department of Obstetrics & Gynecology and Urology Loyola University, Chicago

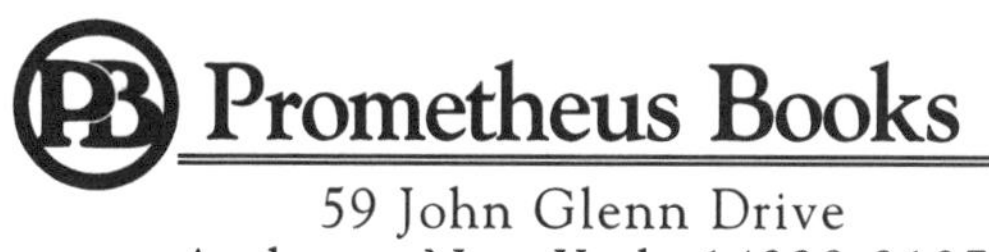

59 John Glenn Drive
Amherst, New York 14228-2197

Published 2003 by Prometheus Books

Inquiries should be addressed to
Prometheus Books
59 John Glenn Drive
Amherst, New York 14228–2197
VOICE: 716–691–0133, ext. 207
FAX: 716–564–2711
WWW.PROMETHEUSBOOKS.COM

07 06 05 04 03 5 4 3 2 1

Library of Congress Cataloging-in-Publication Data

Murphy, Magnus, 1963–
Pelvic health and childbirth : what every woman needs to know / by Magnus Murphy, and Carol L. Wasson : foreword by Linda Brubaker.
p. cm.
Includes bibliographical references and index.
ISBN 1–59102–078–6 (pbk. : alk. paper)
1. Pelvic floor—Diseases. 2. Childbirth. 3. Urogynecology. 4. Natural childbirth—Complications. [DNLM: 1. Genital Diseases, Female—etiology—Popular Works. 2. Delivery, Obstetric—Popular Works. 3. Pelvic Floor—surgery—Popular Works. 4. Urinary Incontinence—etiology—Popular Works. WP 120 M978p 2003] I. Wasson, Carol L. II. Title.

RG482.M87 2003
617.5'5—dc21

2003005896

Printed in the United States on acid-free paper

Contents

Acknowledgments

This book took a long time to come to fruition. When I first perceived the need in the beginning of 1998, the task appeared, (and was) daunting. It took more than four years between that first idea, and the product you now hold in your hand. There have been many disappointments and hard work along the road, but all that pales in light of the excitement of finally seeing the book on the shelves. This is not primarily because it is finally done, but mainly a sigh of relief that the information contained in these pages is finally out there, available to all. I have long believed that information regarding the pelvic floor and its relationship to childbirth is essential for women, newly pregnant women, and older women alike. Public knowledge regarding the long-term dangers of childbirth, as well as incontinence and pelvic organ prolapse specifically, is woefully inadequate.

There are many people whom I would like to thank for their contributions to the birth of this book, many who don't even know what influence they've had. First of all, I'd like to thank my parents who encouraged me to develop independent thinking, as well as my teachers and professors at my alma mater, Stellenbosch University

Medical School in South Africa, for a medical education that is second to none. To the colleagues I've had over the years and especially my current colleagues in Calgary, thank you for everything I've learned and am continually learning from you, even if you don't even know it at the time. To Dr. Linda Brubaker, thank you for your support of the idea, especially at a time when the whole concept looked like a mountain too big to climb. To Carol Wasson, my co-author, I can only say *thank you*. Without you there would have been only a concept. Steven L. Mitchell at Prometheus Books, our editor, also deserves a large thank you for not only guiding us through the final stages, but mostly for being brave enough to take on this (initially) apparently obscure topic from new authors. Steven had the insight to realize that the extent to which the pelvic floor was unknown was the best proof for the need of this book.

I'd like to thank Dr. John Miklos (www.urogynecologychannel.com) for the liberal use of his absolutely gorgeous illustrations. A picture truly is worth a thousand words. Thank you also to Milex Corporation for the illustrations of pessaries and cones.

The individuals from whom I have learned the most, however, have been my patients through the years. You have shaped my thinking to a large extent and have inspired me continuously to do better and to try harder.

Lastly, my family, to Ronel, Michele, and Meghan; thank you for your patience, and accepting the lost family time with understanding. I truly plan to make it up to you . . .

Magnus Murphy

My greatest thanks go to Dr. Magnus Murphy. Thank you for allowing me to be your partner in getting this very important message out to women of all ages. Your patience, sensitivity, caring, and commitment are unparalleled. Next, to our editor, Steven L. Mitchell—thank you for believing in this project. From the very beginning, you gave your time and input. Your direction has been invaluable. To Dr. Linda Brubaker, thank you for your support. You made this happen.

Also thanks to my dear friend and colleague, Suzanne Studinski, I'm sorry I missed all our lunch dates. And to Missy Ainsworth, my assistant, your research skills and organization have always kept me on track.

To my husband, Jim, without you I am nothing. To my daughter, Lea, I know I've missed out on so many moments. I only hope you will let me regain them, as I love you so much. To my mom, Helen, you have been my inspiration for a lifetime. And finally, my utmost respect and appreciation goes to the brave women who have shared their stories with us. In doing so, you have helped so many others.

Carol L. Wasson

Foreword

Dr. Linda Brubaker

Birth is a profound experience and often one of the highlights of a woman's life. Yet, this experience may be impacted by changes in a woman's body, particularly changes in bowel or bladder control. Unfortunately, these changes are rarely discussed among women.

I have provided treatment for many new mothers who wished that they had known pelvic problems could happen following childbirth. Their stories are not necessarily similar. One woman may minimize relatively major symptoms because her "miracle baby" was born safe and sound. Another may deeply regret her decision to delivery vaginally instead of having a repeat Cesarean section. These women share a desire to provide the safest birth environment for the baby, but differ in their tolerance of pelvic symptoms. Clearly more information is needed for modern women.

The authors of this book present this information for consideration, without pushing a predetermined plan for any individual woman. Quite the contrary, it is the woman's individual choices that are of great importance. Each mother-to-be should gather the information that she needs to determine the birth choice that is most appropriate for her. As a physician, I would hope this decision would be based on sound information, not emotions, fear, or untested traditions.

Patients, midwives, and doctors all agree that the perfect birth outcome includes both a healthy infant and a healthy mother. Yet birth, trends and traditional, are being questioned like never before. Women have become assertive in obtaining their health care. Most mothers would willingly transfer risk to themselves if it helped their child in any way. However, if the baby is equally safe, and there are differing risks for the mother, it seems most reasonable that she be given this information. *Pelvic Health and Childbirth* fills this important niche. It is a comprehensive book that provides a great deal of important information for mothers-to-be and new mothers alike. I suspect this book will be the first of many such editions.

It is likely that many readers will pick up this book and respond with strong emotions. I encourage you to read carefully but critically. It is my hope that this book will stimulate discussion, debate, and most importantly scientific advances. Women's health care has been subject to politics and emotions for many years. Perhaps this volume will help turn the tide and expose the pelvic impact of motherhood. When you are finished, consider being part of the solution—part of the positive dialog to improve the health of new mothers.

Dr. Linda Brubaker
Female Pelvic Medicine
Department of Obstetrics and
Gynecology and Urology
Loyola University, Chicago
President of the American Urogynecologic Society

ONE
A Silent Epidemic

Suzanne is a forty-four-year-old mother of three children. The oldest is twenty-six, the next is twenty-five, and the youngest is eight. She started experiencing a bit of incontinence just after her thirtieth birthday. But she resisted slowing down. Her passion for playing softball kept her active, although to hide any embarrassing leakage, she always had to wear a pad during the games. Running became increasingly difficult. At age thirty-six, Suzanne had her last child. She suspected during delivery that her "insides" were not quite right. She pushed as hard as she could even though something somewhere was tearing. In the year that followed, her physical condition worsened. It felt like something was literally falling out of her vagina. Her clothing felt constricted. And any running, jumping, or lifting worsened the incontinence. She never knew when the next accident would happen, so she simply remained at home for days at a time, while depression began to overwhelm her.

This book is not about reassurances. It is about a problem that has been around forever, one that remains hidden and ignored, even though it has assumed epidemic proportions. As with most medical topics, it seems the ability to reassure patients counts most highly.

Understandably, we all like to be told that everything will be all right. But in this book, we intend to alert and inform women as to a very serious health threat—one that is being downplayed and even ignored.

The female pelvic floor is one of the most important organ systems to women's health. Yet many women do not even know that it exists. This is despite the fact that pelvic floor disorders are affecting millions of women of all ages.

The pelvic floor is exactly what its name implies, a floor, specifically the floor of the pelvis, the pelvic organs, and the whole intra-abdominal cavity and all its organs. Like any floor, the pelvic floor provides support and keeps everything above it in its proper place. Without this foundation, the intra-abdominal organs would simply fall through the pelvis.

Pelvic floor dysfunction or damage may result in devastating consequences—ones such as varying degrees of urinary and fecal incontinence, pelvic organ prolapse (a falling in or out of the organs), chronic pelvic pain, and sexual dysfunction. These defects and disorders are directly related to damage during vaginal childbirth.

Many excellent books describe the pregnancy and natural birth experience in detail, offering helpful hints and advice. They focus on the immediate experience, the miracles of pregnancy and giving birth to a new life, reassuring the reader that childbirth is a natural process that usually ends happily with a healthy mother and child. Wonderful as this is, the process of vaginal childbirth has important implications that are often brushed over or not discussed at all. Most pregnancy texts prepare women for a full return to normal urinary and bowel continence functions after only a short period of time. There certainly is little mention of the fact that the pelvic floor might be permanently damaged.

Almost every woman who has experienced vaginal childbirth has sustained some damage to the pelvic floor—ranging from very mild to extremely severe. Many of the effects of this damage are not experienced immediately and may commonly appear years later. Certainly this is one of the reasons why the detrimental effects of vaginal birth have not been adequately discussed between a woman and her doctor. Although it is almost impossible to predict which women will develop pelvic floor damage during childbirth, ignoring the topic is simply unacceptable.

The fact that there is a high risk of pelvic floor injury during childbirth has been known and written about in medical articles since the early part of the twentieth century. Over the last decade, a virtual explosion of scientific articles regarding pelvic floor injury has appeared in respected obstetrical journals. Certain medical conferences consistently shed light into new research and prevention methods. However, it is shocking and surprising that while the academic community is debating these issues, the public's level of knowledge is disturbingly low. There are no lay books on the topic and an almost total disregard of the problem in the current crop of pregnancy and childbirth books. Despite academic acceptance, pelvic floor disorders are, in reality, a silent epidemic. They represent a serious threat to women's health, one that is being minimized for a variety of reasons.

The pelvic floor is one of the most neglected parts of the human body, largely because its function is unseen and unappreciated. Its disorders may be embarrassing to most and definitely are considered an unfit topic for polite conversation. In truth, women cannot easily discuss these problems with friends, family, or even with a physician. Consequently, these disorders have not generated the kind of influence within the medical community that allow for open discussion between patients and physicians. Also, compartmentalized medical specialties have led to fragmented research and neglect in disseminating information to women.

This book will examine the pelvic floor itself and its integral role in childbirth. We will explore the possible effects of vaginal childbirth on the health of this extremely important structure and follow the natural progression of pelvic floor disorders. The most common pelvic floor disorders will be described in detail, followed by a thorough coverage of both surgical and nonsurgical treatments.

It is time to bring these issues to the forefront so that women know there is no need to fear embarrassment, suffer indignities, or alter the quality of life. There are answers and outlets for discussion. And, certainly this book will help women take an informed, proactive role in the medical treatment of a host of pelvic floor disorders.

We will also focus on many of the changes that have occurred in childbirth philosophy over the years. The reasons behind these changes show how they are inspired not only by the desire to improve health, but by motives of political intrigue, economics, and cultural influences.

Finally, the actual facts of cesarean birth will be closely examined. Not only will the technical aspects and benefits of this birthing method be addressed, but also the possible risks and complications for the mother and the newborn baby alike.

However politically incorrect this may be, elective cesarean birth may be one way that a woman can protect her pelvic floor from some of the devastating consequences that may result from vaginal childbirth. Only by being informed about all the risks, as well as the implications of her decision, can a woman make an informed decision about the preferable way to have her baby. We certainly *do not advocate* that all women must undergo a cesarean section, but rather that the pelvic floor as an entity should be discussed with all women and that the risks of pelvic floor damage should be given serious consideration.

The decisions one makes are too often a result of peer pressure, group pressure, and professional pressure about the way it is supposed to be done. We wish to expose the flaws of this thinking and help women better participate in their birthing experience and the decision about how to have a baby, be it by vaginal or cesarean birth. Knowledge about the implications of either decision is essential if a woman is to make not only an informed decision but also her own decision.

Although pregnancy and childbirth are the most common causes of pelvic floor disorders, especially in younger women, there are many other factors that play a role in the development of these disorders. Through this examination, we wish to stimulate an understanding of what women can do to prevent the initial occurrence—or at the very least postpone or mitigate onset—of pelvic floor disorders and their recurrence.

TWO
On the Quality of Life

Pelvic floor disorders can be devastating to the quality of life. Worsening symptoms of urinary and anal incontinence lead to social embarrassment, depression, and even isolation. At the very least, sufferers have a lack of self-esteem and fear the loss of independence. Yet, fewer than half of all women with incontinence seek medical help. Many remain clinically depressed. Often, some experts say, women feel they must accept these conditions as a natural result of childbearing and aging. There is a feeling that nothing can be done about it and, of course, there's the thinking that no one wants to talk about it, so help cannot be found.

Historically, our society, peer pressure, and politics have prevented some women from seeing a bigger picture. Although of the utmost importance, much of the focus in childbirth is on the health of the baby, and on the *immediate* needs of the mother. And certainly, the "natural childbirth movement" has contributed so much in making the pregnancy and childbirth experience happier and more satisfying. But the long-term effects of this short-term thinking are just now being addressed. The issues of pelvic floor disorders are just now coming to the forefront. The question of whether a woman should be able to choose an elective cesarean birth is just now being asked. And, the controversy surrounding this issue is just beginning.

Enter question after question: Do doctors want to perform more cesarean sections for convenience, or because they want to make more money? Why not let nature take its course? Many people have never heard of the pelvic floor. My doctor never mentioned it when I had my first baby, they say. Is ignorance bliss? When will it be acceptable during the childbirth process to focus on the mother's entire lifespan? Are women considered to be selfish if they are concerned about their own long-term welfare during pregnancy and delivery? Are women supposed to simply accept the possibility of significant pelvic floor dysfunction? Since symptoms may only occur years later, is it just *easier* to ignore the whole thing and hope for the best? One might say it's just a fact of life. After all, insurance companies aren't going to pay for elective cesarean sections, so what is the point of this discussion? Nothing is going to change this situation. Put up and shut up, some say. There are no easy answers.

Though, hopefully, when the quality of one's life is truly threatened, an individual will seek change, and avenues for change do exist. There are many places to get help. Although pelvic floor dysfunction is one of the most prevalent yet underreported health care issues, the tide is beginning to turn. Talk to your doctor. No woman is alone in this issue. Talk to others about it. Listen. There are so many women who *need* to tell their stories. Here are just a few of them:

Sharon

This is my story. It seems like I have had this problem forever. When I was thirty-two, I had my first child. After delivery, I realized I had to wear a pad to keep dry. Four years later, I had my second child. Two years after that, I had my third. With each child, the problem kept getting worse. After the third child, I had to wear a pad every day. It started to affect any intimate time I wanted to spend with my husband. When I let myself enjoy our moments together, the bed ended up being wetter than it should have been. My husband was very understanding and said that it didn't bother him. But it bothered me, and I didn't want to let him know just how much. Soon we just stopped having any private time together. Things got to the point where I didn't go out anymore unless it was a social event with the family. During one of these events, my pants got wet after a coughing spell. Even though I was wearing three pads, it was not enough to protect me from embarrassment. That was when I decided to go to the doctor. I went to a walk-in clinic at first, a place where no one would know me. The physician there sent me to a specialist who did not want to talk to me about this problem until I lost weight. I had been fighting the weight battle since my youth. But they told me that it would be hard to operate on me, make an incision, when I am fat. I lived another year with the problem. Then I saw another specialist who told me there was a procedure that would help me, one that would not require an incision. I am not sure what to do. I am very busy, and have problems taking time just for me. But my husband encourages me to have this treatment. He says things will go the right way. So, finally, I am going to get this taken care of. Then maybe I won't be scared to do the things I had enjoyed long ago, like laughing really hard and picking my kids up in public.

Donna

Before my surgery at the age of sixty, my life was one big embarrassing problem. I could never go anywhere without knowing where the bathrooms were. I started walking three to six miles per day, and my problem just increased. So even walking was centered on where bathrooms were. Sometimes I would have "accidents" caused by coughing or sneezing. I usually had to get up two to three times in the night to use the bathroom, and that left me very tired. I wore pads for six-plus years to try to solve the problem. Following surgery, I had absolutely no pain, was up and walking right away, and only had one small problem with voiding. That went away after a few weeks. I don't think about where the bathrooms are anymore and the days of wearing pads are over. I had forgotten how wonderful life could be.

Jill

It all started after the birth of our second child. I couldn't run, skip, or dance without losing control of my bladder. I couldn't play ball with my kids without having an accident. Sneezing and coughing was always the worst, always unexpected, always so embarrassing. I had to rely on pads most days, especially if I had a cold. I couldn't even talk to my husband about this problem. It took me a very long time to have the courage to talk to my doctor. When I did, he recommended a simple surgery that would be fairly painless and would have a short recovery period. It's been three months since the surgery, and I am so pleased with the results. It was the best decision I ever made.

Jeannine

I am twenty-four years old and have two children. Both were delivered vaginally. With the first one, I was in labor for about eighteen hours and almost had to have a C-section. After the birth of my second child, I started having problems with urinary incontinence. I always felt full and bloated. My stomach stayed sore with terrible cramps during my period. My legs ached a lot and sex was just awful, so terribly painful. My OB/GYN said that due to childbirth problems, I had uterine prolapse. In other words, my uterus was falling. When my insurance company would not pay for the recommended surgery, a different type of procedure was ultimately performed. After recovery, all the symptoms went away. But six months later, they all returned. Why? I can't go through this again. I can't work and I can no longer afford to go to the doctor. I don't know what to do.

What Is Natural?

The unfortunate fact is that we simply have no way to determine which women will develop pelvic floor disorders after a vaginal childbirth. Throughout the years, maternity care has changed tremendously, and I believe that an understanding of the pelvic floor and the effects of vaginal childbirth are about to cause a small revolution, at least in certain parts of the first world's population. One thing is certain. The future will bring continual change to maternity care and to women's health care issues overall.

Today many, if not most, pregnancy books on the market are fueling the idea that less is best as far as medical interventions are concerned. So-called natural childbirth has become the "in" phrase, and those who use the term tout vaginal births as the only acceptable outcome except in extreme circumstances. Numerous examples of successful vaginal births in these books describe horrendous labors where the limits of safety are severely tested. In spite of this, these births are hailed as success stories. Prolonged second-stage labor (when the cervix is fully dilated and the mother is pushing) is considered to be of no harm. Any intervention by the obstetrician is regarded as unnecessary meddling that robs the patient of her chance to have a normal vaginal delivery.

Although I believe that many good things have followed from the natural childbirth movement, I also believe that the pelvic floor is natural childbirth's (still unrecognized) Achilles heel. I do agree that in the case of a healthy fetus, a long second stage of labor will not necessarily have any detrimental effect on the baby, but the effects of a prolonged second-stage labor on the mother's future quality of life has been overlooked. Later complications of a vaginal childbirth are no less of a problem, just because they do not occur in the labor room. So what is natural? Many might feel it's natural to care about the long-term quality of life.

THREE
Understanding the Pelvic Floor

A SUPPORT SYSTEM

The pelvic floor is the support structure for the pelvic organs and intra-abdominal organs. Pelvic organs include the uterus, bladder, rectum, and sigmoid colon (part of the large bowel). The intra-abdominal organs, such as the rest of the bowel, lie on top of the pelvic organs. Like any floor, the pelvic floor provides support and keeps everything above it in its proper place. Without this foundation, the intra-abdominal organs would simply fall through the pelvis.

One of the reasons that the pelvic floor fails so often is because, originally, its function was purely urogenital. In other words, it was a mere closure and continence enabler for mostly horizontally placed organs such as the vagina, bladder, and anus/rectum. With the evolutionary development of bipedal or erect posture, the pelvic floor suddenly had to be able to provide support of organs that now lie in a vertical position where they are completely subject to the force of gravity. In the horizontal position these organs were supported by the abdominal wall with its strong muscles, as well as the pubic bone. In the erect posture of humans, there is precious little preventing these organs from falling through the genital openings in the pelvic floor.

However, the pelvic floor is much more than a foundation or floor. It also determines the actual shape and position of the pelvic contents, a shape that is mostly defined by the collagen support tissue of the pelvis, the attachments of this tissue, and by the muscles and ligaments of the pelvic floor and the attachments of these structures to the pelvic bones. Broadly, the pelvic floor can be seen not only as support layers but also as consisting of parts of the organs that transverse through it. In this view, the female pelvic floor would comprise the levator ani muscle, in addition to the endopelvic fascia, ligaments, neural tissue, blood vessels, and parts of the vagina, urethra, rectum, and their sphincters.

Dynamic Involvement in Bodily Functions

Yet the pelvic floor is not a passive support structure, as its name would imply. And it is not an unyielding platform. In reality, the pelvic floor plays a direct, active, integrated and essential part in urination, defecation, sexual function, and childbirth. It is key to the maintenance of urinary and fecal continence, aiding in the integrity of the bladder and rectal storage systems, and in the prevention of inadvertent wetting or soiling. During urination and defecation, its role changes from support and facilitation of continence, to a vital contribution to these activities. For example, the pelvic floor permits the expansion of the lower rectum to allow the passing of feces. For urination, relaxation of the pelvic floor allows the descent of the bladder neck, which causes a funneling of the upper urethra, thus helping to initiate urine flow. The muscles of the pelvic floor play a role in the amazingly intricate control that people normally have over their bowel movements. Not only does it allow gas to escape while it maintains continence of solid and fluid fecal material, but the timing of such relief is under its direct voluntary control in the normal and usual situation.

A Safety Net

An intact pelvic floor prevents prolapse, or a falling of the pelvic organs into or out of the vagina. It prevents a downward bulging of the bladder and an upward bulging of the lower rectum, while preventing the uterus from falling through the vagina. Note that the terms "downward" and "upward" are misleading, and are only geographically correct when a woman is lying in the examination or *lithotomy* position in the gynecologist's office.

It is especially while straining during urination or defecation that the tendency for these organs to bulge into the vagina may become severe, and it is basically only an intact pelvic floor that can prevent that from happening. For this reason, it is important that the pelvic floor examination be performed in the erect position as well. If the examination is only performed with a patient lying down, the physician could easily miss many pelvic floor support problems.

Importance to Sexuality

Positive sexual experiences are some of the most pleasurable human sensations. Healthy sexual relations form the bedrock of long-term relationships and bolster a continuing positive self-image. A normal pelvic floor is necessary for optimal sexual function.

During intercourse, the muscles of the pelvic floor play a major role in orgasm. The contractions of these muscles in the female provide a tighter vaginal grip on the penetrating penis, facilitating male and female pleasuring. During orgasm, the pelvic floor muscles contract in rhythmic waves, which is the main reason for the pulsating nature of any orgasm.

Pelvic floor damage in the sexual context is commonly known as a "stretched" or "lax" vagina. Although for obvious reasons this is seldom presented to their physicians as a problem, affected women and their partners often reveal some dissatisfaction with their sexual lives. It is, of course, not purely the size of the vaginal aperture that matters, just as the size of the penis is not the most important thing. The real problem is often the discomfort associated with genital prolapse, or even incontinence during intercourse. However, it is common for numbers of women to complain that their sexual satisfaction, and that of their partner, has suffered as a result of decreased sensation, presumably caused by vaginal relaxation.

It is also important to note that relaxed vaginal openings can create annoyances caused by air going in and out of the vagina. Many women complain about "popping" sounds during intercourse, and even when simply walking. Presumably this happens as the air gets trapped, is compressed, and then escapes. This seldom, if ever, seems to happen in women without at least some vaginal relaxation.

A Role in Providing Core Strength

The pelvic floor helps to provide core strength to the body, a fact that is not often appreciated. It not only plays a role in stabilizing the pelvic girdle, but it also is an essential part of the mechanism whereby one increases the intra-abdominal pressure to stabilize and splint the abdominal and trunk muscles. It can be understood this way: A sagging pelvic floor would make the generation of intra-abdominal pressure impossible. As any athlete knows, the abdominal muscles are incredibly important for just about any power-requiring muscle action anywhere in the body. And, weak or ineffective abdominal muscles are also one of the most common causes of back pain.

Visualizing the Pelvic Floor

The easiest way to visualize the pelvic floor is to imagine a trampoline (see illustration on page 27). Think of one of those small round-framed trampolines found in many backyards. Now, imagine the frame of the trampoline being slightly bent, so that it is somewhat wider from side to side than from front to back, and that the black canvas (webbing) is sagging. Next, picture three holes cut into the canvas one behind the other. The front hole is the smallest. The other two holes behind it are almost equal in size, but a bit larger than the hole in the front. With this, the pelvic floor picture is almost complete, but a few details still have to be sketched.

In this model of the normal human pelvis the three holes represent the urethra, the vagina, and the rectum, in that order. The

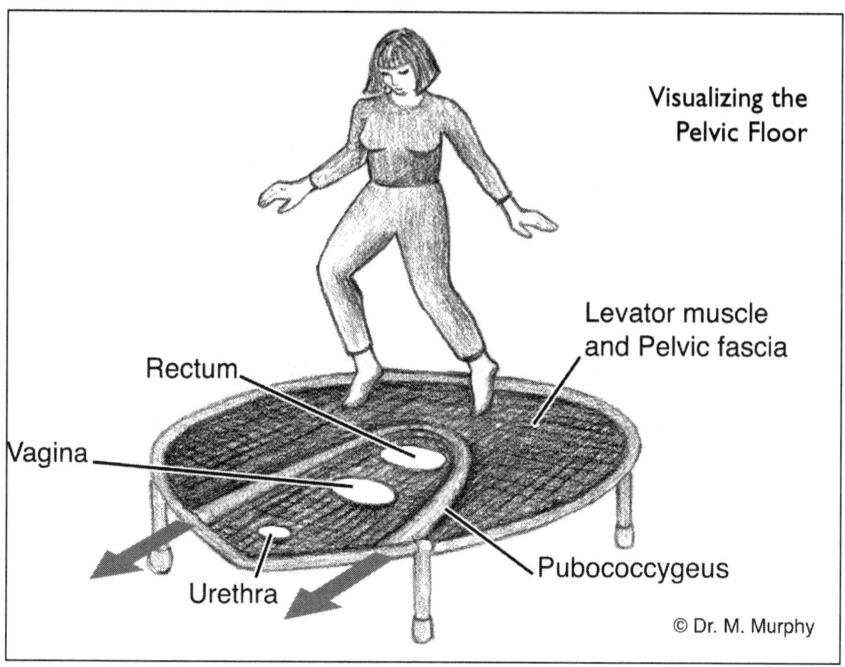

canvas represents the pelvic floor and the frame represents the pelvic bones. In humans the pelvic floor consists of different layers, the most important of which are muscle and fascia layers, to be discussed in detail later on.

In the illustration the pubococcygeus muscle is highlighted. This is a very strong part of the levator ani (pelvic floor) muscle, which forms a loop around the pelvic openings, and has a very important role in closing off these openings and preventing organs from falling through these holes. By looking at the direction of pull of this muscle as illustrated, the concept should be clear.

The pelvic fascia layer is not clearly differentiated from the underlying muscle in our illustration, but it is of cardinal importance. Both the fascia as well as the levator (pelvic floor) muscles need to be attached to the frame of the trampoline (pelvis) to provide "lift" or support to the pelvis. Think of a real trampoline where the webbing is torn from the frame—you would not want to jump on it!

The real pelvic floor is not really horizontal or even flat. Instead, the muscles sometimes form a concave shape, just like our imaginary sagging canvas, but since it is an active organ it can also con-

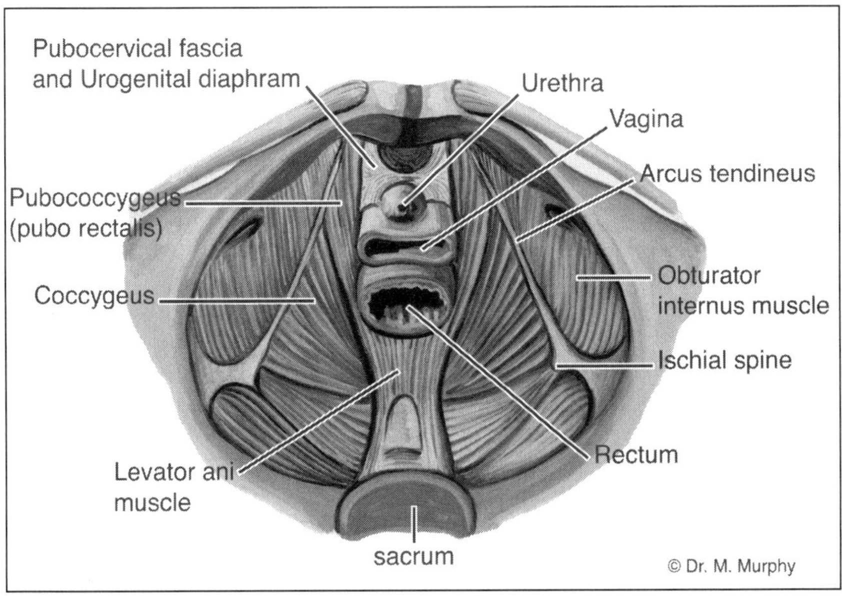

tract into a convex shape, thus creating active lift. Note that most medical students have only seen the collapsed, concave pelvic floors of cadavers; in a live person with a healthy pelvic floor, this image is wrong.

Female Pelvic Floor Muscles

The female pelvis is divided into two compartments, with the lateral attachments of the vagina dividing the two. The front (or anterior) compartment is the urogenital compartment containing the urethra and vagina, and the back (posterior) compartment contains the rectum.

The most important muscles include the pubococcygeus, iliococcygeus, coccygeus, and ischiococcygeus muscles that together form the levator ani muscles (one on each side meeting in the midline). Although considered different muscles, they form a single unit in one plane and function in unison. In reality, the ischiococcygeus muscle consists of only a few muscle fibers on top of the sacrospinous ligament. This ligament has practical implications for one of the commonly performed surgical procedures we will look at later.

The levator ani muscles are mostly made up of fibers of the so-called slow-twitch type. Unlike ordinary skeletal muscle, levator ani muscles do not tire easily and are able to provide constant support and prolonged contraction even though a person may not be aware of it. So we are not usually conscious of levator ani muscles, yet they are also under our voluntary control. Mainly, this is because they also contain "fast-twitch" fibers that allow quick responses to messages from the brain during episodes of involuntary and increased intra-abdominal pressure, as occurs when we cough, sneeze, or laugh. The resultant contraction then serves to counteract the downward pressure that is generated.

There are a few other muscles we should be familiar with if pelvic floor defects are to be understood. These are the various sphincter (clamping) muscles of the tubular hollow organs perforating the pelvic floor and whose dysfunction may cause fecal or urinary incontinence (leakage).

Very basically, both the bladder neck and the lower rectum have strong sphincter muscles, each under voluntary control. This control is needed to overcome sudden urges, to avoid urination, passing gas, or defecation at inappropriate times or under unacceptable circumstances. The sphincter muscles can also contract reflexively, however, to counteract involuntary episodes of increased intra-abdominal pressure. It is obvious that the weakness caused by direct damage to the muscle tissue itself or to its nervous supply will lead to poor function and the danger of incontinence. Everyone is aware, at least, of his or her rectal sphincter muscles. If one does not actively relax this sphincter, as well as part of the levator muscle (the puborectalis), one just cannot defecate. The flip side is immediately obvious. If the rectal sphincter and puborectalis relaxes when it should not, or if it cannot contract or maintain the necessary tonic contraction, because of damage or exhaustion, involuntary defecation or incontinence is a high probability. Sphincter muscles are in effect our safety clamps. They give us control over our bodily functions, and without them we would be at the mercy of every bowel and bladder contraction. This would have made civilization as we know it almost impossible. The sphincters we are concerned with here are under both conscious and involuntary control. This means that we can consciously and purposefully contract them, but that they also have the ability to contract as a reflex reaction without the need for us to consciously think about it. Most sphincters also have constant tone, just like the levator muscles. This means that the sphincter is always contracted under normal conditions. You can easily verify this by feeling the tone in your anal spincter if you try to insert a finger into your anus (provided that your sphincter is intact and working of course).

How Do Pelvic Floor Muscles Work?

For a muscle to work efficiently and properly there are a few basic prerequisites. First, the muscle has to be properly implanted into a strong point from where it can exert traction or tension. Think about a rope that is used to pull something. Obviously, it has to be attached securely at both ends to enable efficient transfer of the forces created. Consider the common problem of an athlete with a torn muscle. A torn pelvic muscle is no different, but the problem is simply more difficult to diagnose.

Second, the muscle needs to be innervated, which will enable it to receive messages from the brain or spinal column. The return loop of the nerves is equally important since nerves have to return information to the spinal column or brain about the status of contraction and the position of the muscle. The brain has to know when to stop the contraction, or how to modify the contraction to exert just the right amount of force. It is amazing to realize the intricate control we have over our muscles under normal conditions. This precondition for effective muscle action is very important, but also quite problematic.

If the levator muscles and pelvic sphincter muscles are not innervated, no amount of exercise will be able to strengthen the muscle. They are paralyzed, plain and simple. In such cases, women who do or attempt to do Kegel's pelvic floor exercises or use devices such as vaginal cones are unfortunately wasting their time. Many women "cheat" unconsciously, by using alternate muscles to accomplish the pelvic squeezing effect. If not taught how to do the exercises correctly, while making sure that they can indeed contract the required muscles, such women might spend months, or even years, fooling themselves and wasting their time.

Convincing patients to do pelvic floor exercises is only half the battle, and it is certainly not enough. Doing exercises correctly is one thing, but *can* they be done? Are the muscles actually intact, attached, and innervated? In some cases, doing electromyography (EMG) studies will help to ascertain the innervation status of particular muscles. Electromyography is a diagnostic test used to measure the electrical activity of muscles, in this case, that of the pelvic floor.

Third, for a muscle to contract effectively, the muscle tissue has to be healthy and free of unnecessary scar formation or connective tissue (nonmuscle tissue that keeps tissues together). Previous surgery or damage from childbirth, for instance, can sometimes lead to repair of the muscle, but with significant scar tissue, something that is not conducive to effective muscle action.

The correlation between damaged, torn, and attenuated (weakened and thinned) muscles and problems with pelvic floor function is stunningly displayed in magnetic resonance imaging (MRI) illustrations shown at the 2001 American Urogynecology Society (AUGS) meeting. After viewing illustrations of both healthy and damaged pelvic floor muscles (specifically levator ani muscles), participants were asked to determine which patients had prolapse, incontinence, or were normal. Those MRI illustrations support the fact that conditions that can cause damage to pelvic floor muscles will be risk factors for developing various disorders—such as prolapse.

FOUR
The Pelvic Fascia

Fascia Acts as Scaffolding

In the illustration in chapter 3, the top of the pelvic muscle trampoline represents the pelvic fascia. Fascial tissue is connective tissue, which is the soft-tissue framework that holds our various body parts together, or apart, depending on their location. Without connective tissue, the body would literally fall apart in separate clumps of muscle, brain, and various specialized tissues that would lack a recognizable form. Combinations of different types of collagen form the connective tissue.

In the pelvis, the fascial layers provide a framework that implants the muscles that encircle the pelvic floor. These layers also surround the various pelvic organs, keeping each in proper place. Fascial layers consist of blood vessels, nerves, and fibrous collagen connective tissue that enclose the pelvic organs and attach each to the pelvic sidewalls. There are separate levels of pelvic floor fascia, each being important for supporting a specific part of the pelvic floor while preventing certain specific problems, ones that may appear if the specific fascia level fails.

The pelvic fascia provides the main support for the uterus and cervix, and lateral support for the vagina. The lateral attachments of both vaginal walls (anterior and posterior) lead to the most important preventative measures against a collapse of the bladder or the bulging of the rectum into the vagina.

Rectovaginal Fascia

In the posterior position, the rectovaginal septum (a septum is basically a fascia layer between two closely related organs) is the most important. It is the fascial layer that separates the vagina from the rectum, preventing the collapse of the front of the rectum wall into the vagina during straining, such as when a bowel movement is passed. The pelvic fascia surrounds each tubular organ as it perforates the pelvic floor, and is also integrally embedded in the wall of each organ, attaching each to the pelvic sidewall. Therefore tears or damage to this fascia can have significant consequences for the normal functions of these organs, their positions, and the strength and integrity of their sidewalls. The rectovaginal fascia has been the subject of much controversy. Only recently has it generally become accepted that there even is such a thing in females. This is particularly interesting since it has always been known to exist in the male.

This rectovaginal septum is currently thought to be important in establishing the integrity of the vaginal and rectal walls. It also anchors the perineal body, the term for the thickened part between the anal and vaginal openings. The perineal body is formed by the insertion of multiple small muscles and strong connective tissue units, including the anchored rectovaginal septum. Most of the muscles involved surround the lower vagina and can be clearly felt during a voluntary contraction when placing two fingers in the lower vagina. The external anal sphincter is also attached to the perineal body. Any disruption or dysfunction which results, for instance, from a tear through this area (which is extremely common during childbirth) could destroy the insertion point of multiple muscles, connective tissue structural units, and the attachment of the rectovaginal septum.

For some unexplained reason, the most commonly performed episiotomies in North America are midline episiotomies. This means that the cuts are made directly downward from the bottom of the vaginal entrance. Of course this means cutting right into the perineal body, which may have severe consequences for the integrity of the wall between the vagina and the rectum. Furthermore, as we now know, an intact insertion is one of the prerequisites for effective muscle action, and damage to this insertion point either by spontaneous tearing or by an episiotomy, could negatively influence their effective action. And, the repair of minor to moderate outlet tears or episiotomies have traditionally been left to some of the most junior members of an obstetrical team. Often, adequate repair of these injuries has not been given proper consideration, resulting in future complications.

A tear in the rectovaginal septum can cause the perineal body to lose its anchor and to fall downward. Its effect will be substantial during episodes of increased intra-abdominal pressure or straining, causing the whole perineum to bulge downward. This downward movement can cause the branches of the pudendal nerves (the main nerves of the pelvic floor muscles) to stretch, potentially leading to further damage that can worsen over time. If these stretching forces become chronic, permanent damage is likely.

Pubocervical Fascia

The pubocervical fascial layer also supports the bladder and the urethra. This layer (which is also densely integrated with the vaginal mucosa) acts as an unyielding "hammock" for the bladder neck, which is essential for urinary continence. Tears of this layer, either centrally or laterally to its attachments at the pelvic sidewall (paravaginal defects), are the most common causes for urinary stress incontinence as well as anterior vaginal prolapse. But this is not only of academic value. Distinction of the site of fascial disruption is crucial for the long-term success of surgical repair.

Relatively recently, a new understanding of pelvic floor support, stemming from the above new information, has led to a paradigm shift in thinking regarding pelvic organ prolapse and incontinence. During a clinical examination, the gynecologist will be looking to see if a specific site of fascia or ligament rupture can be identified. This will then allow the doctor to plan a site-specific repair, resulting in a much higher long-term success rate. Such repairs can also be

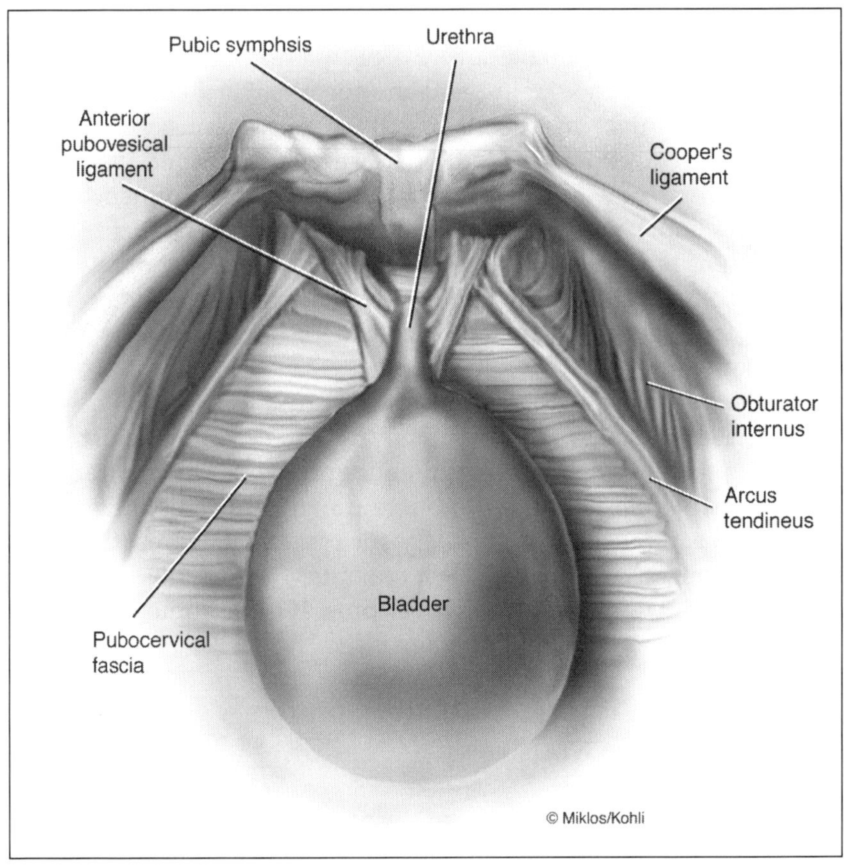

performed as much less invasive procedures with quicker recoveries and less morbidity (negative side effects). Unfortunately, too many vaginal surgeons, both gynecologists and urologists, still understand the pelvic floor under the paradigm that was developed at the beginning of the previous century. This "one-shoe-fits-all" understanding does not allow for individual variations, with the effect that everyone gets the same operation. Given the poor understanding that has been the norm, the success rates achieved are quite remarkable.

In the absence of adequate muscular support to the pelvic and abdominal contents, the full brunt of their weight and pressure falls on the fascial layers. In cases of muscular atrophy (weakening from loss of bulk), or injury or weakness from other reasons, this fascial layer has the burdensome task of providing the only support. Unfor-

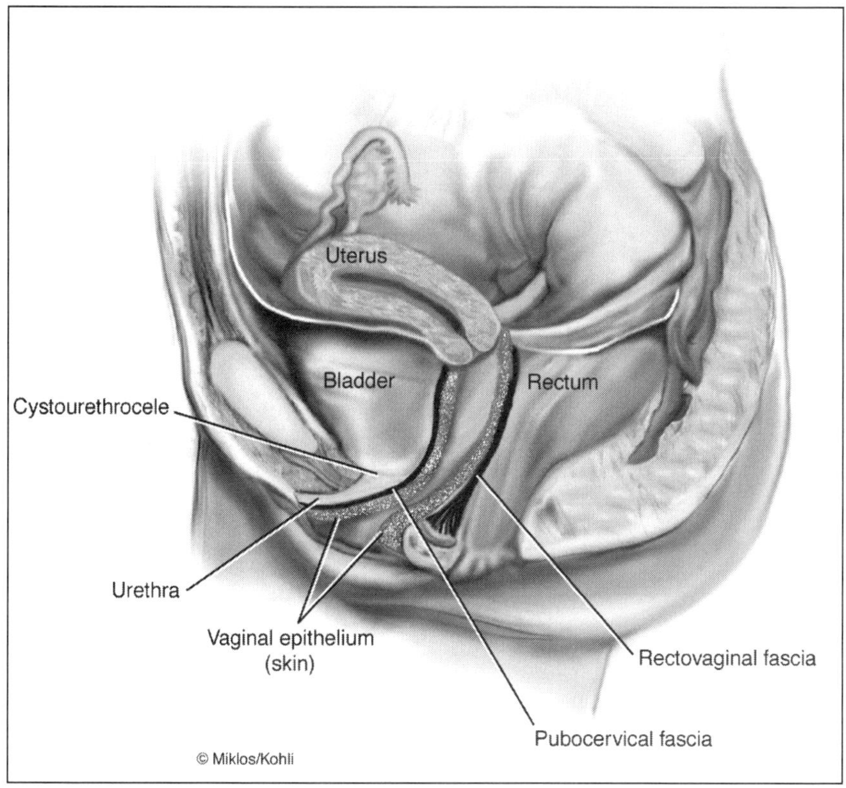

tunately, some of the same causes of muscle and pelvic nerve deterioration also cause tears or stretching of the fascia. Even if initially intact, in the absence of the pelvic floor muscle support, the fascial layer will continue to stretch out over time or eventually tear. Chronic conditions such as straining at the stool, obesity, lifestyle, occupational issues, and the final insult to the female pelvic floor—menopause—eventually contribute to a failure of the pelvic fascial support layers.

Fascia and Genetics

Certain inherited disorders of connective tissue cause a propensity toward hernias and other tissue support problems. It is a well-known fact that patients with genetically determined abnormal connective tissue, for instance those with Ehlers-Danlos or Marfan syn-

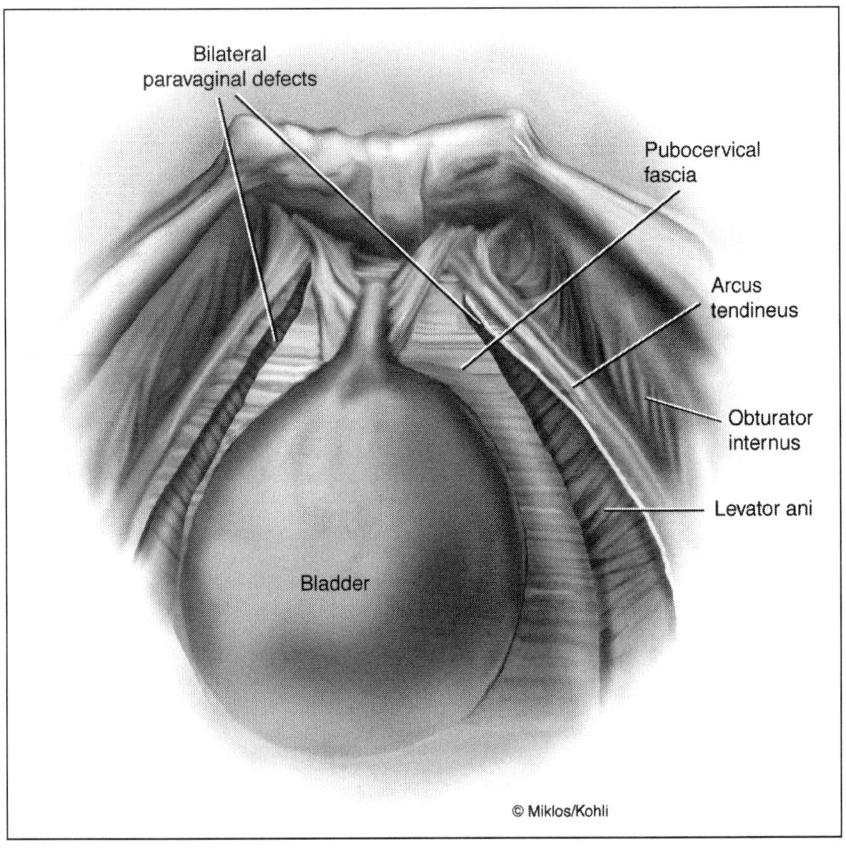

drome (see glossary), have increased rates of pelvic organ prolapse. So, it is probably safe to state that there is a range of genetically determined connective tissue disorders, which might be prognostic (predictive) of future problems. Some of these might be unrecognized as yet, or variants of the norm, and not clinically obvious. Nevertheless, I believe the future holds the possibility of testing a patient's individual susceptibility to connective tissue disorders by checking their genetically determined connective tissue health. Unfortunately that is not yet possible.

Numerous authors and researchers suggest that there might be racially based differences in connective tissue strength, possibly related to differences in the collagen type mix in the connective tissues of the various races. It is known from experience that pelvic prolapse is more common in certain races, but I have yet to see a large study confirming this, or a definitive explanation for this phenomenon. But it is my belief that genetically determined differences will indeed be found.

It is also clear that there is a familial nature to pelvic floor problems. This is easy to understand if a genetic basis for connective tissue strength is postulated. Weak connective tissue is genetically determined, and as a result it makes perfect sense that these problems do seem to run in families. The problems are so common, however, that this is not really a helpful finding as yet.

Fascia and Hormones

An interesting theory about acquired pelvic fascia weakness is that it is hormone dependent and, specifically, estrogen dependent. It is well known that many of the urogenital tissues (see glossary) are extremely sensitive to estrogens and rapidly become weaker in its absence, as in the postmenopausal phase. The theory states that a deficiency in estrogen will lead to a change in the composition of the connective tissue (collagen) types that form the pelvic fascia. Thus a strong collagen type would be displaced by a weaker type, which is then unable to provide the support needed. Secondary prolapse and other problems might, as a result, develop with time. It follows then that hormone replacement therapy has a useful role to play in the prevention and possible improvement of such disorders. It is also believed that some of the muscles of the pelvic floor are also sensitive to estrogen and are negatively influenced by its absence or by lowered estrogen levels. Moreover, estrogen deficiency leads to decreased vascularization (blood flow) to the urethra and to decreased co-aptation of the urethral walls. This means that the internal walls of the urethra will press less tightly together, leading to urinary leakage. The atrophy and decreased vascularization lead to the thinning of the interior walls of the urethra, with urinary leakage as the unfortunate result. Although estrogen deficiency is a common contributing factor, it would seldom be the sole cause for incontinence in the absence of pelvic floor weakness, and estrogen therapy in isolation has not been found to be very effective for urinary incontinence.

Progesterone and relaxin are additional female hormones affecting the health of fascia. Progesterone is the hormone that is secreted by the ovaries after ovulation to prepare the endometrial lining (lining of the uterus) for implantation by the embryo. This occurs every month in ovulating women during the latter half of the menstrual cycle, with a tremendous rise in progesterone levels when pregnancy ensues. The placenta eventually takes over the production of progesterone for the duration of the pregnancy, which in turn supports the placenta and causes changes in the mother's body to prepare her for pregnancy and delivery. The fetus (in this case, the placental half of the fetal-placental duet) has to do some work, too! If no pregnancy occurs, a drop in progesterone levels signals the onset of menstrual bleeding.

Relaxin is a placental hormone encountered only in pregnancy. Progesterone and especially relaxin cause laxity in the body's ligaments, and also in other tissues such as smooth muscle. The relaxation in smooth muscle causes dilatation (stretching) of maternal ureters (the kidney tubes moving urine from the kidneys to the bladder) as well as the bowel. This leads to a higher tendency to develop urinary infections, stones in pregnancy, or changes in bowel function. These "relaxation" changes during pregnancy are important adaptations attempting to make the birth process easier. Stretching of ligaments lead to a slightly increased size of the bony pelvis, but unfortunately the flip side is increased instability of most joints in the body. This is one of the causes of lower back pain, sacroiliac joint pain, and a higher risk of spraining knee or ankle ligaments during pregnancy. It is not only joint ligaments that experience change, but also fascial tissue in other body areas, for instance the pelvis. This stimulated the recent finding that pregnancy per se negatively influences the pelvic floor, especially urinary continence. The negative effect of the pregnancy hormones on the integrity and strength of the pelvic fascia could lead to its increased tendency to stretch, tear, or incur damage during pregnancy and delivery. This finding has led to many debates regarding the contribution of the pregnancy itself versus the route of delivery to the onset of urinary incontinence. This weakness of ligaments and connective tissue during and immediately after pregnancy might be one more important reason to refrain from activities such as heavy lifting or any other activity that significantly strains the pelvic floor during pregnancy and for about six weeks after birth. No bodybuilding until six weeks after delivery!

Fascia, Chronic Straining, Obesity, and Smoking

As we know, the pelvic fascia is susceptible to stretching and tearing. This commonly happens during childbirth. Unlike the muscles shown in the pelvic trampoline illustration, the pelvic fascia cannot bounce back to its normal shape. This is a result of its particular collagen composition. And, no amount of exercise can restore it to its former condition. Further causes of fascia damage include chronic straining during heavy lifting, chronic lung disease which causes chronic coughing (including smoking, which also decreases estrogen levels), or chronic constipation with repeated and constant straining in attempts to evacuate the bowel. As will be seen later, chronic straining from constipation can potentially lead to pelvic muscle damage too, but by another route. Obesity causes increased strain on the pelvic tissues for obvious reasons.

Fascia and Vitamins

Another well-known cause for connective tissue weakness is vitamin deficiencies, especially a lack of vitamin C. It is conceivable that subclinical nutritional disorders could lead to degradation of the body's connective tissue, contributing to genital prolapse and the other pelvic disorders. Also interesting is whether nutritional disorders, such as those found in many young women, might not through vitamin deficiencies lead to later connective tissue and pelvic floor disorders.

FIVE
Pelvic Nerve Injuries

Jeannette, a thirty-three-year-old mother of three, has undergone nineteen procedures to correct pelvic floor damage. Vaginal delivery impaired the nerves that controlled her bladder, leaving her incontinent and without feeling in her bowel. "I was wearing diapers for two and a half years. It's ironic that I don't have a C-section scar, because I have scars down my spine and right side of my bottom, and seven scars in front, all from trying to correct childbirth injuries," she said in an interview with the *Wall Street Journal.*

Muscles can function only if they are innervated. Damage to nerves can take many forms, not necessarily being permanent or complete. Nerves can be damaged by overstretching, by being crushed against a hard object (for instance a bony point), or by tearing or being cut during an episiotomy, perhaps. If the nerve is not completely severed, the term used is "neuropraxia." Such injuries can usually repair themselves in time, although often deficits remain. More severe injuries can lead to the death of nerve fibers and subsequent dysfunction of the particular muscle innervated by that nerve fiber. As we know, effective muscle action requires that the nerve supply be intact. Without this essential element, muscles degenerate and waste away or atrophy. The same is true for muscles that are not used for other reasons. Just think of someone whose leg is in a cast, or consider the effects of weightlessness on the muscles of space station inhabitants.

During vaginal childbirth there are multiple possibilities for nerve damage within the pelvic area. From the descent of the fetus's head through the pelvis, the pelvic nerve plexuses (see glossary) and individual nerves are compressed against the bony pelvis. One of the very important nerves that supply the pelvic floor is the pudendal nerve. It is very vulnerable to a combination of crushing and stretching forces. These nerves, one on each side, supply most of the voluntary muscles of the pelvic floor and perineum and are essential to normal pelvic muscle action. Within their course through the pelvis, they angle sharply around bony points called the ischial spines. The Latin root of the words "ischial spine" can be translated as "thorn of the hip joint." The ischial spines (again, one on each side) are part of the ischial bones, of which there are two. These are the lateral (side) bones of the pelvis. Since the interspinal distance is the narrowest part of the midpelvis, the fetal head invariably applies significant force to the pudendal nerves in these areas. Since the nerves are relatively unable to move because of their sharp angulation around these bony points, they are especially vulnerable to crushing, stretching, and tearing.

Many medical researchers have proven, beyond a reasonable doubt, that pelvic nerve injuries are extremely common during vaginal childbirth. It was found that the percentage of women who develop nerve injuries is as high as *60* to *80 percent*. This was found in women who gave birth vaginally or in women who had emergency cesarean sections after they had reached the second stage of labor. A cervix that is fully opened with the fetal head ready to come out defines the second stage of labor. During this stage the mother is usually actively pushing, the fetal head is deep in the pelvis, and the vagina as well as the pelvic muscles and fascial layers are maximally stretched. All the factors to cause compression and shearing forces on the pelvic nerves are in play.

Although most of the injuries improve partially or completely in time (pudendal nerve recovery could take up to a year), pudendal nerve injuries have been found to be cumulative with successive vaginal deliveries, leading to altered continence sometimes many years later. This is in contrast to the mechanical injuries sustained by the anal sphincter, which has been found to be maximal during the first vaginal delivery. In contrast to cesarean sections performed after the patient had been in active labor, no pudendal nerve injuries are found after elective cesarean section prior to labor.

The pudendal nerves are, in addition to the functions already mentioned, the main nerves of the pelvic organ sphincter muscles (a voluntary component). These, mainly, include the external anal sphincter, the bladder neck sphincter, and certain small muscles surrounding the lower part of the vagina. Other nerves that might be damaged include the sympathetic and parasympathetic nerve chains, and together this can lead to the dysfunction and weakening of the levator ani muscles, which are a crucial part of the pelvic floor.

Researchers have found no pudendal nerve damage after elective cesarean births. With elective cesarean births, the fetal head is usually still high in the pelvis, or even above the pelvis, and the tremendous compression and stretching forces have not been applied. Some recent studies have indicated the possibility of a loss of the protective effect of cesarean births on the incidence of urinary incontinence after three cesarean sections. These findings did not include any mention of deterioration of the protective effect on anal incontinence or pelvic organ prolapse. The speculation is that there might be cumulative disruption of some pelvic nerves (specific ones have not been clarified) during successive cesareans. It also seems to be related more to urgency urinary incontinence than to stress incontinence. I believe that the successive effects of manipulating the bladder, and dissecting the bladder downward, off the lower segment of the uterus and upper vagina in the area of the bladder neck during cesarean section, may be the cause. This action may compromise the small nerve branches supplying the sphincter muscle of the urethra, leading to progressive dysfunction of the urethral sphincter, or of the bladder itself with successive cesareans. If this were indeed the mechanism, it would make sense that the protective effect on the other parts of pelvic floor integrity would remain. Of course there are other possibilities as well. It could be the cumulative negative effect of pregnancy itself that outweighed the protective effect of cesareans, rather than any negative effect of cumulative cesarean section. We do know that pregnancy and elective cesarean births do not lead to abnormal pudendal nerve function, by contrast to vaginal delivery.

We certainly don't have all the answers yet. Women who are motivated to choose cesarean birth mainly as a protection of the pelvic floor should keep these uncertainties in mind. At this time I would suggest that given the increasing complications and risks of successive cesareans, elective prophylactic cesarean section with pelvic floor protection as an indication, makes the most sense for women planning a maximum of two children (see section on risks of cesarean birth in chapter 18).

Operative Vaginal Deliveries and Nerve Damage

It is well accepted that operative vaginal delivery carries the potential risk for pelvic damage, particularly with a forceps delivery. The vacuum extractor is associated with a lower risk for this complication. Although some studies have also found the vacuum extractor to be a risk factor for pelvic floor damage, the overwhelming majority indicates little excess risk over and above that of spontaneous vaginal delivery. This is in contrast to forceps delivery, which been found in almost every study to be a significant risk factor for almost all aspects of pelvic floor damage. This includes urinary incontinence, pelvic organ prolapse, and anal incontinence.

Due to this accumulating evidence, a paradigm shift is developing in modern obstetrics. Intervention in pregnancy became very common during the first half of this century and the reasons for this are complex. Some of these reasons have already been discussed in the section on the history of obstetrical management. Others involved the significant status of a few high-profile individuals whose opinions had power to sway the whole medical establishment. The idea of prophylactic forceps delivery was touted as a way to reduce the second stage of labor, and thereby reducing the damage to the pelvic floor. In the same way episiotomy was promoted, these ideas were advanced without the backing of any science. Considering that evidence-based medicine is a relatively new development, we now know that both forceps deliveries and episiotomies are risk factors for pelvic floor damage. Since this realization has taken hold, forceps deliveries have been slowly decreasing. Rotational forceps and high forceps deliveries are rarely performed anymore. New obstetrics residents are not being trained to do them, and that will inevitably lead to their demise. Now, the vacuum extractor is more popular. And, obstetricians are shying away from difficult midforceps or trial of forceps deliveries. Performed when a successful operative vaginal delivery is in doubt, trial of forceps deliveries are done in the operating room with the patient ready for an immediate cesarean section and an operating and anesthetic team on standby.

I predict that most forceps deliveries, except for easy outlet forceps deliveries, will soon be a thing of the past.

The level of operative vaginal delivery is determined by the position of the fetal head. For high operative interventions the fetal head is obviously high in the pelvis, midway in the pelvis for mid-operative deliveries and so on, with the head almost out and bulging through the vulva for outlet deliveries. The dilemma is that these operative procedures may be essential to expedite delivery, or to make vaginal delivery possible at all. In cases where labor has already reached the second stage (often after prolonged pushing), it may often be too late to affect the protection of the pelvic floor through a cesarean section over an operative vaginal delivery. As mentioned, some of this damage heals with enough time. Yet there are disturbing studies showing that significant nerve damage persists in a large percentage of women after vaginal delivery. The pelvic fascia can usually overcome the resultant weakness in the levator ani muscles for only a short time. Of course, this is true only if the fascia is intact and attached to begin with. With aging, natural processes and the increasing stretching of the fascia under the influence of the intra-abdominal weight it now solely has to bear, the fascia eventually cannot support its burden effectively and prolapse develops. This can manifest as overt genital prolapse, or urinary or fecal incontinence. Weak sphincter muscles usually lead to incontinence problems. Sphincter defects can arise from the above-mentioned neurological damage or from more direct damage.

SIX
Pelvic Floor Disorders and Childbirth
An Overview

Pelvic floor disorders include urinary incontinence, anal incontinence, pelvic organ prolapse, abnormalities of the lower urinary tract, defecatory dysfunction, sexual dysfunction, and several chronic pain syndromes. The National Institutes of Health (NIH) maintains that at least one-third of adult women are affected by at least one of these conditions. NIH statistics show that 30 to 40 percent of women suffer from some degree of incontinence in their lifetime, and that almost 10 percent of women will undergo surgery for urinary incontinence or pelvic organ prolapse. Interestingly, they say, 30 percent of those undergoing surgery will have at least two surgeries in trying to correct the problem. It is estimated that a half million surgical procedures for prolapse are performed annually in the United States, almost twice as many as procedures performed for urinary incontinence.

The NIH states that although radical pelvic surgery and radiation may provoke pelvic floor dysfunction, the major inciting factor for the development of pelvic floor dysfunction in women is vaginal delivery. The NIH concludes that with the steady increase in the population of older women, the national cost burden related to pelvic floor disorders is enormous in terms of lost productivity, decreased quality of life, and direct health care costs.

In its 2001 annual report, the Pacific Coast Obstetrical and Gynecological Society estimates that the demand for services to care for female pelvic floor disorders will increase by 45 percent over the next thirty years. "We can only speculate on how the impact of increased direct-to-consumer advertising and demystifying of taboo subjects such as urinary incontinence and pelvic organ prolapse will add pressure to the demand," say its authors, adding that afflicted baby boomers will be a more vocal and proactive group than their predecessors. Furthermore, the report uncovers that more than half of the women seeking care are aged thirty to sixty years, a fact that is important for health care policy makers, as well as health care programs, they say, because women in this age group may be working full-time inside and outside the home. They maintain active lifestyles and are also savvy consumers of health care and will seek out and demand the best treatment of their problems.

The Relationship Between Pelvic Floor Disorders and Childbirth

What follows is a brief overview of that relationship. Although not fully outlined here, each issue mentioned will be defined and discussed in detail within the remaining chapters in this book.

Pregnancy itself has been found to have a negative effect on the pelvic floor integrity. This can be readily understood if one considers the effects of the specific hormones that are elevated in pregnancy. Elevated levels of the two hormones progesterone and relaxin, specifically, can lead to weakening of collagenous tissues throughout the body. These hormones not only have effects on the placenta and uterus, but also on many other tissues in the body. Some of

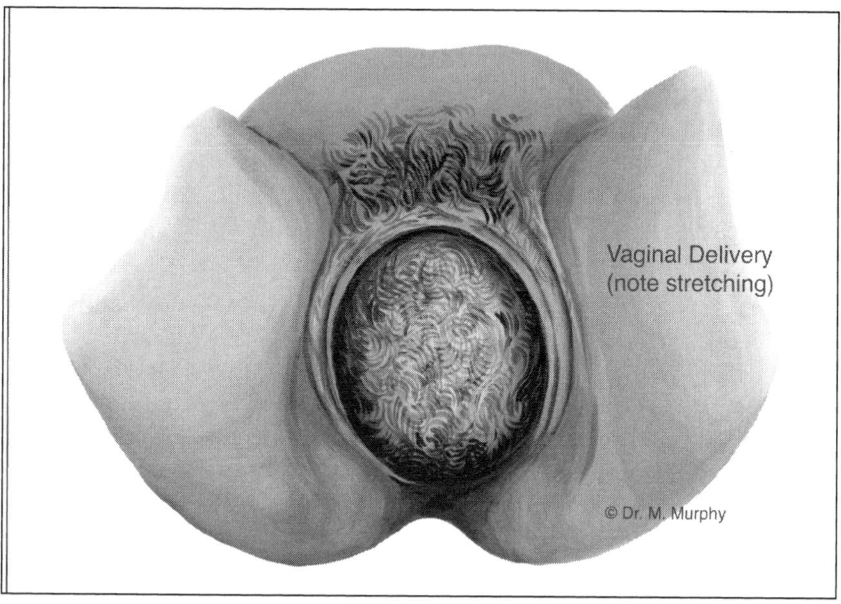

these effects include dilatation (distention) of some blood vessels that can then cause blood pressure changes, which can often lead to the common problem of feeling faint in pregnancy. The softening effect of these hormones that causes the distention of blood vessels also leads to the softening of ligaments throughout the body. This can lead to greater mobility in joints, including those of the pelvis, which leads to slight increases in the diameter of the birth canal. They also play a role in the softening of the cervix immediately before and during labor. Unfortunately, the global effects of these hormones also have negative results. These include back pain, an increased tendency for joint strains, and for the purpose of our discussion, increased problems with urinary incontinence.

These hormones also affect the collagenous tissue of the pelvis, which leads to weakening of the support structures of the vagina, bladder, and rectum. Usually, hormonal changes after pregnancy lead to progressive strengthening of these support tissues with an improvement in symptoms.

Unfortunately, the vaginal delivery process can lead to further injury and weakening of the pelvic floor through various mechanisms, some of which are permanent. They include tearing or stretching of the anterior urethral ligaments, lateral vaginal fascia attachments, damage to the pubocervical fascia or rectovaginal fascia, or damage to the apical (highest level of the vagina) fascia support of the vagina and/or uterus. In fact, damage to connective tissue could form a continuum with greater or lesser degrees of damage along the whole length of the vagina.

Vaginal delivery is not only related to fascia and connective tissue tearing and damage, but also to injury to pelvic nerves, sphincters, and muscles. It is well known that the first vaginal delivery is the most important risk factor for mechanical injury to the anal sphincter muscles. Pelvic nerves, specifically the pudendal nerve, are damaged progressively by successive vaginal deliveries. These vaginal births, quite likely considered successful and uncomplicated at the time, may lead to severe incontinence problems later.

The incidence of anal sphincter injuries tearing during the first vaginal delivery is frightening. Up to one-third of women have been found to have anal sphincter injury after the first vaginal delivery. Fortunately most of these are asymptomatic even though damage might be seen on an ultrasound. Recognized third-degree tears of the rectal sphincter (complete tear of the sphincter) occur in up to 2 percent of women, with up to a 43 percent incidence of some long-term anal incontinence problems afterward.

The most common injury found is mechanical injury to the anal sphincter muscles, but other injuries include nerve and pelvic floor muscle injuries. These injuries are clearly the result of the delivery, rather than the pregnancy per se.

Women with altered anal continence, however, have about a 90 percent chance of recognizable anal sphincter defects. As a result of the higher risk of future anal sphincter damage with successive babies after a previous injury, as well as the increased likelihood of severe symptoms and poor prognosis, increasing numbers of obstetricians and almost all urogynecologists (specialists in pelvic floor dysfunction) recommend cesarean section for subsequent deliveries.

Instrumental vaginal delivery, specifically forceps delivery, has been found to be a high risk for the mechanical injuries described above. There is less evidence to indicate that vacuum operative vaginal deliveries cause the same problems. As far as the vacuum is concerned, I believe that the risk will depend not only on the instrument, but also on the operator. During a normal vaginal delivery the vaginal outlet tissues have some more time to stretch. This is one reason for allowing the mother to push more naturally (in a panting manner) rather than according to the "medical" model, where she "has" to push for ten seconds or some arbitrary length of time, every time. Such long pushes generate increased expulsive forces and although it possibly leads to shorter second stages and quicker deliveries, it might lead to more perineal damage as a result of a sudden expulsion of the fetal head without sufficient stretching of the perineum. Sometimes however, such pushing is the only way to "get the baby out," and is strongly encouraged almost universally. Vacuum (and forceps even more so) leads to just such a fast delivery, and I think this contributes to the damage observed.

Perineal damage is classified into four degrees. A first-degree tear involves only the vaginal mucosa, with no involvement of underlying muscle. Second-degree tears involve underlying muscle, but do not involve the external rectal sphincter. Third-degree tears usually involve a transection of the external rectal sphincter. Fourth-degree involves a tear through the vaginal mucosa, the perineal muscles, the external rectal sphincter, and the internal rectal sphincter and rectal mucosa, thus creating an open wound between the vagina and the rectum.

Notes on Episiotomy

Episiotomy was originally introduced with good intentions, and a strong belief that it would help to protect the pelvic floor against damage sustained during childbirth. This belief was rational on the basis of shortening the second stage, thereby shortening the time of compressive forces in the pelvis, attempting to prevent uncontrolled perineal tears, and the expectation that a "clean cut" surgical incision would heal better than torn tissue. Unfortunately, this did not turn out to be the reality. In fact, not a single proposed benefit of episiotomy has been confirmed, except for anterior vaginal tears, which are usually of no consequence anyway. By contrast, it has been found that episiotomy may actually increase the chances of a severe perineal and vaginal laceration. Postdelivery anal incontinence rates are higher after midline episiotomy, which is unfortunately still the most commonly performed episiotomy in North America. Also, the incisions have not been found to heal any better than spontaneous tearing. Another downside to consider is this: If an episiotomy is done, the woman ends up with a 100 percent chance for a vaginal wound, which per definition is at least comparable to a second-degree laceration. Episiotomy always involves underlying perineal muscles. If episiotomy is not performed, there is always a chance of no sustained tearing, or only superficial grade-one tearing. As mentioned, episiotomy has not been found to significantly reduce the risk of higher-order tears.

Having stated this, which can be supported by medical literature, there are times when episiotomy is totally appropriate. Individualization is the key. It is *universal* episiotomy, as was practiced in the past, that is wrong.

SEVEN
Understanding Urinary Incontinence

Urinary incontinence affects at least 15 million people in the United States alone, of whom 85 percent are women. Over the lifespan, statistics show that women are twice as likely as men to have urinary incontinence, and where younger adults are concerned, its prevalence in younger women is seven times higher than that of younger men. The direct cost of treating incontinent women exceeds $16 billion per year. The indirect costs to society such as loss of productivity and the costs of incontinence products is unknown, but carries a significant economic impact.

Although it is assumed that the prevalence of urinary incontinence increases with age, it should not be considered a normal part of the aging process. Some studies demonstrate minimal increases in prevalence with age, and an even higher prevalence in younger age groups. A study that included women between the ages of twenty and eighty years reported an overall prevalence for urinary incontinence at 53.2 percent. Even in younger women, ages twenty to forty-nine, the figure tops 47 percent, and as we have said, fewer than half of these women seek treatment. Some fear further embarrassment, some fear surgery, and many feel that it's simply their lot in life. Others feel their problem is insignificant, as symptoms might be occasional, for instance occurring only during a severe cold. However, the great tragedy is that a large number of women are inhibited from participating in activities they enjoy or must do on a daily basis. Among the major problems reported by these women were lack of self-esteem, fear of smell, embarrassment, sexual difficulty, and loss of social contact and productivity.

One of the clearest indications as to the prevalence of incontinence is the feminine hygiene market. This is a rapidly growing market characterized by a wide range of dryness products, drugs, and other therapies, estimated at more than $10 billion in total sales annually in the United States, most of which is not covered by insurance. Every day, one encounters television ads for urinary moisture protection, all targeted to women. Walk around the shelves of your neighborhood pharmacy and it's abundantly clear that incontinence means huge profits. Any way you look at it, incontinence is big business.

Incontinence and Pregnancy

Up to 4 percent of women who have never had children complain of occasional urinary loss. During pregnancy, the percentage increases to 9 percent at sixteen weeks gestation, and 40 percent beyond thirty-four weeks gestation and through six to eight weeks after delivery. Although most recover, approximately 15 percent continue to experience problems. The big question for our purposes is how many women will encounter future urinary incontinence problems that are directly related to damage from a past vaginal birth.

The most important obstetrical risk factors known to possibly contribute to postpartum urinary incontinence are:

- a first vaginal delivery
- a prolonged second stage
- a forceps delivery

- episiotomy
- obesity
- epidural anesthetic on the basis of a prolonged second stage
- a third-degree perineal tear
- fetal weight more than 9 pounds (4 kg)
- high maternal age at delivery
- cigarette smoking

TYPES OF URINARY INCONTINENCE

Understanding urinary incontinence can be difficult as there are different types of incontinence. Not all types of incontinence are related to pelvic floor damage. The most common type is *stress urinary incontinence* (also called genuine stress urinary incontinence), which is usually a consequence of pelvic floor dysfunction. The other main type of incontinence is *urgency incontinence*, or what is referred to as an overactive bladder, stemming from bladder muscle instability.

Unfortunately, women are at much higher risk than men for the development of urinary incontinence. This is not only related to childbirth, but also in some degree, to the short urethra in the female and its anatomical relationship to the vagina.

Normal bladder function involves the storage of urine volume in the bladder at low pressure. A normal bladder wall and muscle will allow stretching to store up to 14 fluid ounces (400 ml) of urine without significant increase in the pressure inside the bladder. During this filling phase, the pressure inside the urethra, at the level of the bladder neck specifically, will be higher than the pressure inside the bladder, even during physical activities such as coughing, sneezing, or jumping. The prevention of urine leakage is the job of the urethral sphincter and the backboard support of the pelvic floor fascia, onto which the urethra gets compressed if intra-abdominal pressure increases. Damage to either the backboard support (damaged fascia or pelvic floor muscles) or a weak urethral sphincter will cause an inability to sustain the required higher pressure in the urethra. During episodes where the pressure equalizes, or where the bladder pressure exceeds the urethral pressure, urinary leakage (incontinence) will occur.

This dysfunction is easy to understand through the following analogy: Imagine laying your garden hose on soft mud with the tap open. When stepping on the hose, it will simply sink deeper into the mud while the water will continue to flow. If the same hose is lying on your driveway, stepping on it will stop the flow. The unyielding driveway creates the backstop against which the hose is compressed. In the pelvis, the fascia performs this function, provided it is intact.

Increased bladder pressure can also be generated by contraction of the bladder muscle itself. Normally, bladder muscle contraction should only occur during active and voluntary voiding, and should be associated with urethral sphincter relaxation. A lack of coordination between the bladder muscle (detrusor) and urethral sphincter will lead to abnormal voiding or incontinence.

THE INCONTINENCE PARADIGM

The two types of incontinence, stress urinary incontinence and urgency incontinence (detrusor instability), have been formalized into two distinct types by the International Continence Society's (ICS) classification system. Almost universally accepted, this classification has guided the understanding and treatment of incontinence since the 1970s.

The problem with this classification is that a large number of patients fall into both categories or suffer from *mixed* incontinence. The classification suggests a plan of pelvic floor exercises, behavioral modification, or surgery as treatment for stress urinary incontinence. For urgency incontinence, recommended treatment is via medication only, with surgery an unlikely necessity.

The dilemma of patients with significant stress incontinence, but severe detrusor instability has been a big problem. Many of these patients have been denied surgery for fear of doing the "wrong" thing.

The new *integral theory* may be a way out of this dilemma. This theory attempts to correlate most incontinence symptoms to pelvic floor dysfunction and damage, allowing the possibility of overcoming the reigning confusion and offering renewed hope for patients that are currently not being helped. Only time will tell if the promise will be realized. (Of course there are other causes of incontinence and those will be described briefly later.)

But for the most part, the classical ICS paradigm still rules.

Therefore much of what we discuss on urinary incontinence will fall back on those viewpoints, recommendations, and interpretations.

GENUINE STRESS URINARY INCONTINENCE

The word "genuine" indicates that the diagnosis has been confirmed. This is often accomplished by specialized tests called urodynamic assessment. In the latest classification of the International Continence Society, such a confirmed diagnosis of stress urinary incontinence is also called "urodynamic stress urinary incontinence." The typical case history of a patient with genuine stress urinary incontinence is that of a squirt of urine occurring in the event of increased intra-abdominal pressure when coughing, sneezing, laughing, running, or lifting. The fact that the great majority of women suffering from this are either pregnant, or have had vaginal childbirth, has been known since early times. Consider that in 1919, Howard A. Kelly, the first professor of gynecology at the Johns Hopkins Medical School, co-authored a text entitled *Disease of the Kidney, Ureters, and Bladder*. He wrote:

> The commonest form of incontinence is the result of childbirth, entailing an injury to the neck of the bladder; it is occasionally seen in the elderly nullipara and is most common after the age of 40. It is usually progressive, beginning with an occasional dribble, later becoming more frequent and occurring on slight provocation. In its incipiency, a strain, cough, sneeze or stepping up to get on a tram car starts a little spurt of urine which, in the course of time, initiates the act which empties the bladder.

Most studies cite a high incidence of urinary incontinence in pregnancy in healthy young women even during the first pregnancy. Prevalence rates as high as 50 percent are reported. Most of these women recover urine control after the pregnancy, but not all. Unfortunately, a great many of those who recover control have sustained sufficient pelvic floor damage, enough to predict renewed urinary incontinence, with or without genital prolapse and anal incontinence. While successive pregnancies, and especially successive vaginal deliveries, are associated with recurring urinary incontinence, their effect has not been as significant in cases of anal damage or incontinence.

The natural progression of stress urinary incontinence is from mere leakage to eventual continuous, constant wetness. This progression is related to progressive dysfunction or damage not only of pelvic support, but also of the internal urethral sphincter and urethral ligament support. Another possible cause of constant wetness is vesicovaginal fistula, which will be mentioned later.

Stress incontinence is usually treated by correcting the anatomical deficiency, whether by a conservative method or by surgery.

URGENCY INCONTINENCE

In this chapter, the terms "bladder instability" and "bladder overactivity" are used interchangeably. Although the International Continence Society has discarded the term bladder "instability" in favor of "overactivity," many physicians are still using the former terminology. Taking a personal look at urgency incontinence, or what is commonly called an "overactive bladder," women describe it as "having to go *right* now." An overactive bladder also involves symptoms of frequency or having to go very often. Triggers may include hearing water running, feeling cold water on your hands, or seeing a washroom. Though very often there are no triggers with symptoms occurring unexpectedly.

Typically, urgency incontinence occurs after a rise in pressure inside the bladder related to a bladder muscle contraction. Simplistically, it is abnormal for the pressure inside the bladder to rise except when purposely voiding. Such abnormal pressure increases could be the result of bladder instability.

Bladder instability (the medical term is *detrusor instability*) means that the bladder muscle contracts when it is not supposed to. Under normal circumstances the bladder has the ability to distend enormously without any increase in pressure inside the bladder. This occurs as a result of passive distention without the occurrence of any bladder muscle contractions. A person with a normal bladder will still be comfortable with a full bladder, although she will be aware of it intermittently. However, the person with bladder instability suffers from an intense need to urinate even with a small amount of urine in the bladder. This condition may also result from infection or interstitial cystitis (a relatively common urological condition), or may also be caused by diabetes or other medical or neurological diseases. Very commonly, though, no obvious cause is found.

Medication is the usual treatment for urgency incontinence caused by bladder instability. There are some powerful medications on the market, such as anticholinergic agents, that are very effective in many patients. This means that the medication interferes with the cholinergic system, one of the neurotransmitters utilized by the nervous system. These cholinergic neurotransmitters are utilized in smooth muscle stimulation by the autonomic nervous system. The desired effect of using these anticholinergic medications is a relaxation of the bladder smooth muscle. Note that none of these medications work exclusively on the bladder muscle, having at least some effect on other smooth muscle areas in the body. This accounts for many of the side effects, such as having a dry mouth. Another is the possibility of increased eyeball pressure of people suffering from narrow-angle glaucoma, which, as a result, is a contraindication for using these medications.

Diagnostics and Treatment: A Complex Issue

Regrettably, it is often impossible to determine which type of incontinence is predominant without further testing, since patients' histories alone are notoriously inaccurate. As mentioned, patients may suffer from both stress and urgency incontinence, making it difficult to determine which therapeutic approach would be most effective. Obvious pelvic floor prolapse, especially a prolapse of the bladder into the vagina (called "cystocele"), together with urine leakage during coughing, make genuine stress incontinence the likely diagnosis. But according to the ICS classical paradigm, one needs to verify the absence of significant bladder muscle instability prior to offering surgery. Further information can be obtained from a cystometrogram, or more sophisticated urodynamic studies that involve measuring the pressures inside the bladder while filling it with sterile water, for example.

More sophisticated cystometrogram instruments also measure contractions of the pelvic floor muscles and the bladder sphincters, as well as the pressure differentials between the bladder, the urethra, and the intra-abdominal cavity. The main purpose of a cystometrogram is to diagnose or exclude bladder instability, a necessary determination before choosing the therapeutic approach. It is important to rule out bladder instability as surgery, in the setting of bladder instability, could increase the instability.

But seemingly in contradiction, the presence of bladder instability does not necessarily contraindicate surgery. In explanation, one of the worst mistakes a surgeon can make (according to the classical paradigm) is to attempt surgical treatment on a patient who has only bladder instability. Surgery in this setting is unlikely to benefit the patient and, ironically, can lead to a significant increase in the problem. With pure or genuine stress incontinence (in the absence of bladder instability), surgery does have a definite role to play.

More complicated are the cases where both types of incontinence occur together. It is well known that bladder instability can sometimes be caused by pelvic floor damage and the resulting abnormal position of the bladder base. In such cases, surgery often cures not only the stress incontinence, but also the bladder instability. It is a highly unpredictable outcome, nonetheless, and there is a risk that the instability will persist or increase postoperatively. A better understanding of the exact nature of the damage might help researchers to design surgical procedures that can be tailored to a specific defect.

Fortunately, postoperative instability is commonly transient. There are strong drugs available that suppress abnormal bladder muscle contractions, usually leading to significant improvement. Yet it must be noted that postoperative instability is a potential complication that might render a technically perfect operation a failure from the patient's viewpoint, since she is still wet. Certainly, it matters little to her if it is because of "stress" or "urgency" incontinence.

URINARY INCONTINENCE AND THE PELVIC FLOOR

Genuine stress incontinence is usually a result of pelvic floor defects. Although the normal control mechanisms of urinary continence are very complicated, understanding of the main concepts involved is necessary to appreciate the importance of the intact pelvic floor.

The urinary bladder is basically a reservoir. It is a sack lined with an impenetrable membrane and surrounded by a strong muscle called the detrusor muscle. The outflow tube of this sack is the urethra, approximately 1.5 to 2 inches in length. The junction between the urethra and the bladder is called the bladder neck area. A relatively sharp angle is formed between these two, which is important in continence control. A strong sphincter muscle (clamp) surrounds the bladder neck area and is under voluntary control. By contrast, the bladder muscle itself is not under voluntary control, but is carefully regulated by a special center in the spinal column called the micturition (urination) center. The brain does have some control over the micturition center, which gives one the ability to postpone urination until it is convenient. The normal position of the bladder is immediately on top of the vagina and lower part of the uterus, whereas the urethra lies on the lower part of the vaginal roof and is integrally associated with, and attached to, the top vaginal wall.

The pelvic fascia surrounds the urethra and the vagina, and is suspended from the pelvic sidewalls (see illustrations on page 64). This creates suspension support for the urethra, the vaginal roof (also called the anterior or upper vaginal wall), the bladder neck, and the bladder. The integrity of the pelvic fascia, the anterior vaginal wall, and the pelvic musculature is essential to maintain the normal position of the urethra, the bladder neck, and the bladder. There also are ligaments suspending the urethra from the pubic bone in front of it—the pubourethral ligaments. This understanding and the recognition of its importance, has already led to a breakthrough in surgical procedures (see TVT operation in chapter 9). It is clear that even the smallest change in our understanding of the pelvic floor, and especially its normal support and function, can lead to almost revolutionary ideas and concepts.

Continence is provided by a variety of finely balanced factors, which include the position of the bladder neck, the bladder neck sphincters and ligaments, parts of the levator ani muscles, compression of the urethra, and characteristics of the internal urethra. The bladder neck contains an involuntary internal sphincter and a voluntary external sphincter. These sphincter muscles, as all other muscles, depend on the above-mentioned factors for their effective action. Damage to pelvic fascia or pelvic innervation seriously and negatively affects their action. These muscles are the ones we contract to consciously stop the urine stream, doing so by constricting the urethra. During this squeezing action, most of the pelvic voluntary muscles are also contracting, including the levator ani muscles, the rectal sphincter, and certain small muscles surrounding the opening of the vagina.

The position of the bladder neck is extremely important. To recap, there is an angle between the bladder and the urethra. During coughing, sneezing, etc., intra-abdominal pressure is increased as well as the angle between the bladder and urethra, effectively kinking the urethra the way we would bend a garden hose to stop the flow. With an intact pelvic floor and fascia, there is very little sagging in the anterior vaginal wall; therefore, increased pressure on the urethra (transmitted from the abdomen) compresses it against this unyielding floor or backboard and prevents leakage. This effect can be explained once again by imagining a garden hose lying in soft mud. Stepping on the hose will cause it to sink deeper into the mud, but the water will still be flowing through it, since it will not be obstructed. If the same hose is lying on your cement driveway

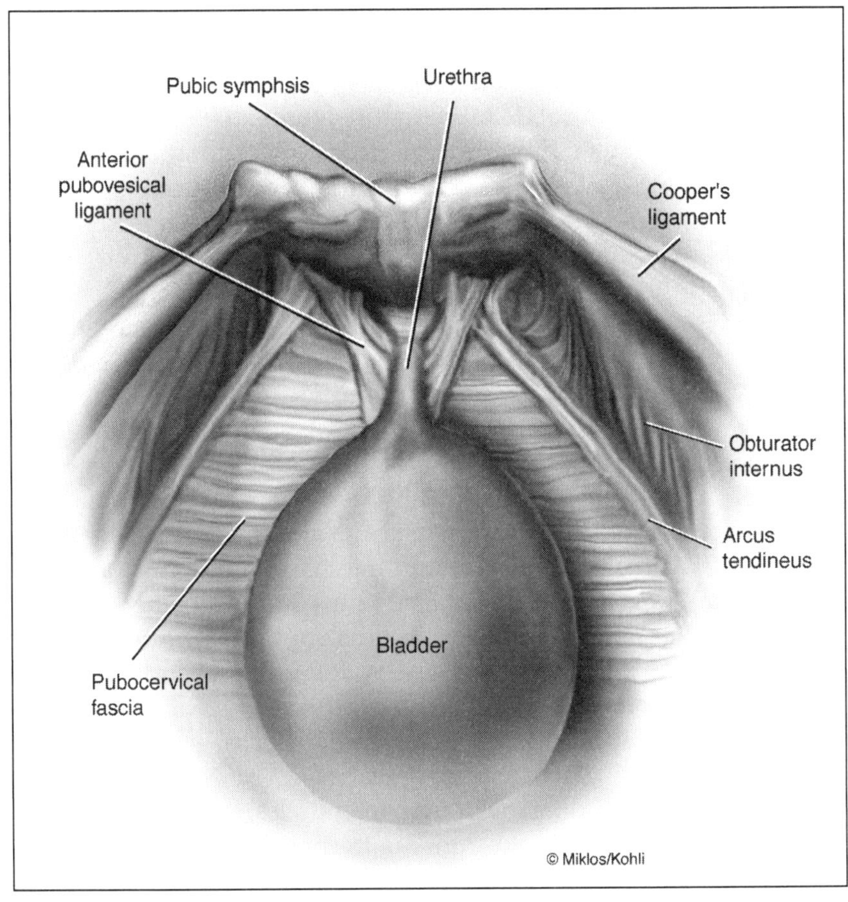

and is stepped upon, it is obstructed and the flow of water ceases. So, the backboard support is extremely important.

The internal structure of the urethra also helps to prevent urine leakage. The mucosal lining fits tightly together and helps to prevent initiation of urine flow. With aging, and as estrogen levels fall, this lining fits together less tightly, contributing to the problem.

Internal urethral deficiencies can lead to stress urinary incontinence. Such deficiencies are commonly called ISD (internal sphincter deficiency). This diagnosis is usually made only by sophisticated urodynamic examination, but can often be inferred from history and an adequate physical examination. Such a diagnosis has implications for the specific surgical procedure that is most likely to provide a cure.

Urinary Incontinence and Vaginal Delivery

Vaginal delivery increases the bladder neck descent and decreases the ability of the pelvic muscles to elevate the urethra and the bladder base. During episodes of increased abdominal pressure, for instance during straining, the bladder neck is lower in women after vaginal delivery, compared to women who have not had children or women who have had elective cesarean sections. It was found that this positional change occurs in more than 50 percent of women after vaginal delivery and is usually persistent. On the other hand, in patients who had elective cesarean births there is almost no difference. It has also been found that the urogenital hiatus (the pelvic opening between the levator muscles and pelvic fascia, through which the pelvic organs course) is larger in women after vaginal delivery compared to during pregnancy, but smaller in women after an elective cesarean than during pregnancy. This could be explained by the fact that pregnancy per se increases the size of this aperture by methods already mentioned, with further negative effects from vaginal delivery but no negative effects from elective cesarean. Presumably, postdelivery reparative processes of the urogenital hiatus cannot overcome the effects of pregnancy plus vaginal delivery to get back to normal, whereas after an elective cesarean the prepregnancy state is achieved. Damage to the pelvic floor with urethral detachment (remember the pubourethral ligaments) was already

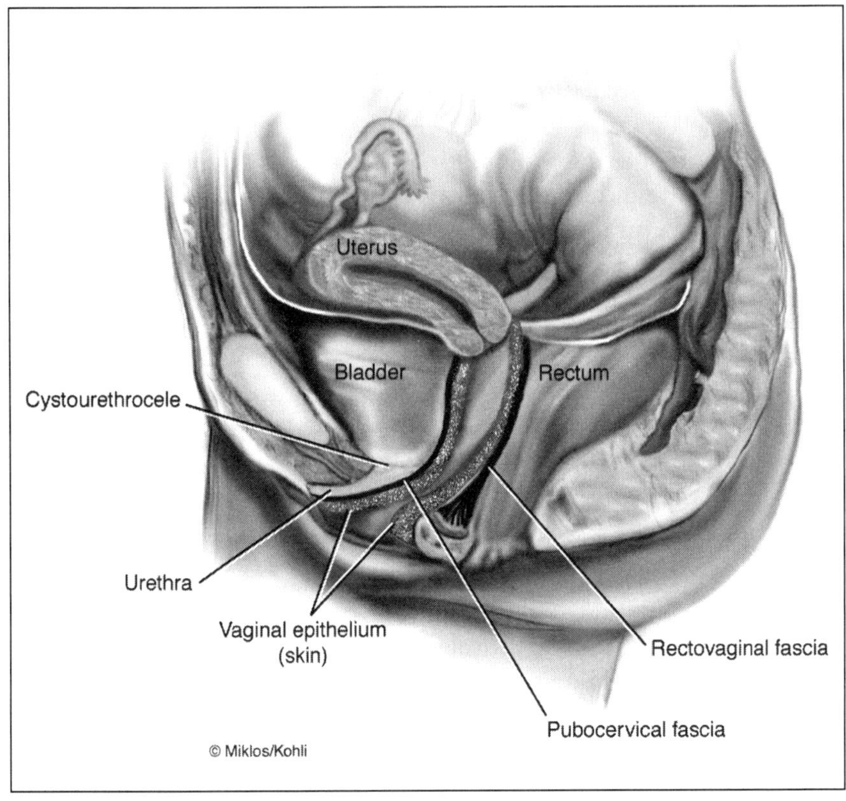

described in 1945, and at that time it was estimated to occur in one-third of patients. It is now known that the very first vaginal delivery can cause damage not only to the pelvic floor muscles and fascia, but also to the innervation of the muscles, and in particular to branches of the pudendal nerve. Further deliveries are thought to add to this risk, although the contributory effect of subsequent deliveries is thought to be considerably smaller than the first. It is a well-known fact that subsequent births are usually easier than the first one. This makes sense considering the uterine muscles have a "memory" of childbirth and since a subsequent fetus will have less difficulty moving downward. This, of course, is the result of decreased pelvic muscle tone and generally relaxed and stretched vaginal tissues and fascia, resulting from the first birth. Unfortunately it turns out that there is a price to be paid for that subsequent "easier" delivery.

The Odds Ratio (a statistical entity calculating the probability of something occurring, and used frequently in medicine) for vaginal childbirth as a risk for urinary incontinence is calculated by some to be 11.15. This means that women have an *eleven-fold* increased risk for developing urinary incontinence after vaginal childbirth over women who have not had vaginal births. Other studies have found widely differing rates, and no current consensus exists about whether the pregnancy itself or the delivery per se has the most profound effect on urinary continence. Most recent studies have indicated an odds ratio of about 3 (threefold increase) of urinary incontinence after vaginal delivery compared with no vaginal delivery. It is interesting that this effect is most noticeable in younger women, since the effects of aging and other chronic conditions become more important in the elderly. Some studies have found a small increased effect of cesarean on urinary incontinence, which could be an indication of the effect of pregnancy per se, rather than the cesarean. In all studies though, cesarean was significantly protective, when compared with vaginal delivery. However, given all the secondary markers for pelvic floor damage directly resulting from vaginal delivery, I don't think there is any doubt that vaginal delivery itself increases the risk, regardless of other factors. Yet it is not clear how big that increased risk is, just that there is a cumulative increased risk with subsequent deliveries.

Every birth attendant has probably had the following experience: a particularly difficult second stage of labor with slow progress followed by a sudden downward movement of the fetal head, and subsequent immediate delivery. I have personally experienced this many times, often in association with instrumental vaginal delivery, possibly just because that allows for more direct sensation. I have gotten the impression that there was a sudden "give" of maternal tissue, immediately preceding the sudden fetal downward movement. It is my belief that many of these situations actually constitute the result of sudden maternal fascia tears, particularly paravaginal fascia detachment. In many of these cases, one can see significant anterior vaginal descent immediately after the delivery. This is just my personal impression, and I have never seen any study attempting to correlate this kind of event with future prognosis regarding incontinence or pelvic organ prolapse. But it is my belief that not only can the maternal tissues stretch or get progressively damaged, but that this can happen in an instant.

Other Causes of Urinary Incontinence

Some other types of urinary incontinence include overflow incontinence, true incontinence, functional incontinence, and other usually temporary and reversible types of urinary incontinence.

Overflow incontinence is defined as the involuntary loss of urine associated with overdistention of the bladder. In most cases this is a result of outflow tract (urethral) obstruction or detrusor underactivity. Therefore, overactive or underactive bladder muscle can lead to urinary incontinence. Fortunately, complete outflow tract obstruction is relatively uncommon in women, but it is sometimes caused by surgery for genuine stress incontinence. Partial outflow obstruction can occur as a result of damage to the higher (level 1) and posterior support of the vagina. Such damage leads to a downward rolling motion of the bladder against the urethra, as well as failure of the bladder neck to open during voiding.

Causes of detrusor underactivity (also called detrusor atony), include such medical conditions as diabetes, thyroid disease, diseases of the bladder nerves, certain medications, alcohol, and infections. In such cases, treatment could take on the form of changing or discontinuing the offending medications, if indeed that is the problem. If outflow obstruction were the result of anatomical and correctable pelvic floor abnormalities, the obvious answer would involve correction of this. In some cases, however, the only effective treatment is a self-catheterization program. This involves the insertion of a small sterile catheter through the urethra into the bladder by the patient herself, usually approximately every four hours. Although it sounds frightening, it is not really all that difficult or uncomfortable and is an easily learned procedure. The biggest problem is for a patient to get used to the idea. Intermittent self-catheterization in the right patient could make the difference from being wet all the time to being dry. Unfortunately some patients are physically or mentally unable to perform the procedure and in such patients the options become much more complicated. Although not within the scope of the book, other options include a permanent indwelling catheter, various kinds of bladder augmentation surgeries, or the surgical formation of a new bladder using resected loops of bowel. These *new* or *neo* bladders can then be made to drain into a stomach pouch (like a colostomy), or into the sigmoid and rectum. In a patient with normal anal continence, the continence mechanism could be sufficient to provide for urinary continence in this way. Obvious potential complications include recurrent infections, electrolyte disturbances, and diarrhea.

True Incontinence

True urinary incontinence is the result of a hole between a urine-containing organ and the outside. Usually this means a hole in the bladder with a tract into the vagina (remember the vagina and bladder are separated by only a few layers), but could also involve the ureter (tube that brings the urine from the kidney to the bladder) or urethra. With modern obstetric management in Western countries this is fortunately rare, but in the past obstructive labor commonly led to such fistulas (holes) causing permanent urinary leakage. In First-World countries, the most common causes of fistulas in the urinary system include pelvic surgery or radiation treatment for cancer. Vesicovaginal (bladder-to-vagina) fistulas are commonly the result of hysterectomy. A single stitch that caught the edge of the bladder could be enough to cause a fistula. Gynecologists who perform pelvic surgery will probably encounter this complication in patients over the course of their career, sometimes more than once, depending on what kind of surgery they perform. The treatment of fistulas that do not heal spontaneously with bladder drainage is always surgical, a topic outside the scope of this book.

Functional Incontinence

Functional incontinence occurs when a person with a normal urinary tract is unable or unwilling to reach the toilet to urinate. This could be because of old age, injuries, or mental problems. Other transient causes include delirium, atrophic vaginitis (thin vaginal skin as a result of a lack of estrogen), medication, and psychiatric disorders.

Nurses Can Make a Difference

RN Magazine (March 1989) states that often nurses are the first ones to hone in on patients' problems with incontinence. They are in an excellent position to help patients escape isolation and stigma. Nurses are encouraged to express a positive attitude by emphasizing that incontinence is common and that many of its causes are curable. Patients should be encouraged to seek further medical advice.

In its guidelines on urinary incontinence (UI), the Agency for Health Care Policy and Research (AHCPR), lists key questions that should be asked in evaluating UI patients. As many UI sufferers are unwilling to seek medical help, the questions below have been formulated to help medical personnel, especially nurses, identify and encourage persons who have the disorder to seek medical treatment.

1. Do you leak urine when you cough, laugh, lift something, or sneeze? How often?
2. Do you ever leak urine when you have a strong urge on the way to the bathroom? How often?
3. How frequently do you empty your bladder during the day?
4. How many times do you get up to urinate after going to sleep? Is it the urge to urinate that wakes you up?
5. Do you ever leak urine during sex?
6. Do you wear pads that protect you from leakage? How often do you have to change them?
7. Do you ever find urine on your pads or clothes and were unaware of when the leakage occurred?
8. Does it hurt when you urinate?
9. Do you ever feel that you are unable to completely empty your bladder?

The answer to the first question helps to identify the symptoms of stress incontinence; answers to questions two through seven assess the severity of urine loss and can also help diagnose bladder instability (overactive bladder); and responses to the last two questions may help identify an outlet obstruction, interstitial cystitis, or urinary tract infection.

EIGHT

Nonsurgical Treatment Options for Stress Urinary Incontinence

In the United States, a recent study by the Public Health Service's Agency for Health Care Policy and Research (AHCPR), a government-sponsored panel of nurses, doctors, allied health professionals, and consumers, concludes that as many as 80 percent of UI patients can be treated or cured. The study maintains that while some patients may be helped by bladder training and pelvic muscle exercises, others may require medication and surgery. The AHCPR guidelines indicate that of the three treatment categories—behavioral, pharmacological, and surgical—that the least invasive behavioral methods should (where appropriate) be utilized first. Behavioral methods include physical therapies such as pelvic floor muscle exercises, with or without the use of vaginal cones, biofeedback, and electrical stimulation—all methods we will discuss in this chapter.

As the primary focus of this book is the treatment and prevention of pelvic floor damage, for the most part I will discuss only those treatments and prevention strategies for genuine stress urinary incontinence. Successful treatment depends upon an accurate diagnosis. Special tests may be required to make the correct diagnosis, as there is often a confusing mix of different causes of urinary incontinence. The following list is a sampling of possible tests that might be performed:

1. **Physical examination:** Includes a gynecological examination and basic neurological examination.

2. **Q-tip test:** A simple Q-tip is placed in the patient's urethra, and the deviation with straining is observed. If the Q-tip deviates more than 30 degrees from the horizontal plane, with the patient lying on her back in the lithotomy position, the urethra is usually considered to be "hypermobile." This could have implications for the treatment offered.

3. **Cystoscopy**: A cystoscope is placed through the urethra into the patient's bladder and the inside of the bladder is observed. Foreign objects, for instance suture material from a previous surgical procedure, bladder stones, infection, interstitial cystitis, bladder cancer, or other tumors can be visualized. A fluid is utilized to distend and fill the bladder. At the end of the procedure, patients are often asked to cough to demonstrate stress urinary incontinence if present. A uroflow study may also be done after cystoscopy.

4. **Postvoid residual volume:** The volume of urine present in the bladder immediately after voiding is called the postvoid residual. This is a particularly important test, since a large volume might indicate either obstruction or abnormal bladder muscle functioning (for instance an atonic bladder, which is a very weakly contracting bladder).

5. **Uroflowmetry:** Uroflow studies are performed by having the patient void into a container that has a sensitive measuring device. The

maximum flow rate, the total voiding time to emptying, and the voided volume are measured and displayed on graphs. Uroflowmetry assesses utility. Although outflow obstruction is much more common in men, uroflowmetry is especially important in women who might have some degree of obstruction after past anti-incontinence surgery.

6. **Pressure-flow studies:** These involve the simultaneous recording of bladder pressure and flow rate. The measured parameters are intravesical pressure (pressure inside bladder), and intra-abdominal pressure. These are measured by catheters, or transducers placed in both the bladder and rectum.

7. **Intravenous urography (pyelography):** Intravenous dye is injected, and abdominal X rays are taken. The dye is excreted by the kidneys and they, as well as the ureters, can be seen. This test is useful for the detection of uterovaginal fistulae, which are sometimes related to pelvic surgery. Sometimes it is utilized to confirm ureteric patency.

8. **Voiding cystourethrography:** This is the simplest contrast radiological study for the evaluation of the lower urinary tract. Contrast is placed into the bladder, usually transurethrally, after which fluoroscopy (X rays) is utilized while the patient voids. This test provides images of some anatomical features including the bladder outline, the position of the bladder neck, the position of the urethra, and often the presence of urethral diverticula.

9. **Urodynamic Assessment: Two Different Tests May be Used to Test the Bladder:**

   a. Simple cystometrogram: A cystometrogram is a test where the pressure inside the bladder is measured. In its simplest form, a catheter is placed in the bladder, connected with a fluid column where the meniscus can be read against a measuring tape. Increasing pressure inside the bladder would elevate the meniscus, which can be directly observed. The change in height is then the change in pressure. The measured pressure corresponds to the pressure inside the bladder, added to the intra-abdominal pressure, which is exerted on the bladder from the outside. To obtain pressures inside the bladder alone, the intra-abdominal pressure needs to be subtracted. For this, multichannel urodynamics is required.

b. Multichannel urodynamics: These more sophisticated tests utilize various catheters to measure pressures in different body cavities. Pressures are usually taken from inside the bladder, as well as inside the rectum (which corresponds to the intra-abdominal pressure), and often inside the urethra as well. Computerized manipulation of the data can yield results very specifically isolating certain organs and their particular pressures.

10. **Electromyography:** Electrodes are often placed on specific areas, specifically the anus and perineal area, but in more sophisticated tests specific sphincters and muscles can be isolated with electrodes to pick up the electrical impulses of sphincter activity. Not only the presense or absence, but also the strength and timing of muscle/sphincter contractions to other happenings in the pelvis can be measured.

11. **Videourodynamics:** This is the investigation of choice for complex cases, especially in the presence of neurological disease, or after previous complex surgical procedures have failed to correct the problem. Videourodynamics encompass multichannel urodynamic testing including fluoroscopy. Radio opaque dye is used for the filling medium during the urodynamic assessment, and fluoroscopy is utilized just like in voiding cystourethrography. The combination of measured pressures and volumes, as well as direct visualization of the anatomic landmarks and changes in positions and forms, yields a wealth of information that can be combined for diagnostic purposes.

12. **Ultrasonography:** Ultrasound is widely used in gynecology. It is safe, relatively simple, and can yield a lot of information regarding the bladder, urethra, and the pelvic floor.

13. **MRI:** So far MRI studies have been used only for experimental and study purposes (as far as urogynecology is concerned). As a result of the superior anatomical discrimination, MRI is slowly becoming a more commonly utilized technique for imaging of the pelvic floor for various disorders.

This is not an exhaustive list as there are currently a large number of possible tests to investigate the function of the pelvic floor, and to quantify and specify the nature of the problem. Next, we'll cover some of the prevention and treatment strategies for urinary incontinence.

Obesity and Smoking

Stress incontinence is associated with pressure differences between the bladder and the urethra. Anything that increases this pressure difference will tend to increase the problem. Logically, obesity, with extra weight on the bladder, will only make the problem worse. Some patients can achieve dramatic improvement in their problem by losing weight. Severe stress incontinence greatly curtails physical activity, which of course makes the weight-loss endeavor so much more difficult.

Another lifestyle issue that has to be dealt with at the outset is the smoking habit. Smoking lowers estrogen levels in the body, and it also leads to chronic coughing. There you have it—another good reason to butt out.

Medication

Medication plays a small role in the treatment of genuine stress incontinence. Since the problem is anatomical in most cases, medication does not lead to much improvement. In cases of bladder instability camouflaged as stress incontinence (yes, that happens), medical therapy is the right choice. This situation can occur if the primary trigger for an abnormal bladder contraction is not the usual visual or auditory stimulus, but something like a cough. The leakage is thus a result of the bladder contraction and not from abnormal pressure distribution as in genuine stress incontinence. If the contraction occurs soon enough after the trigger, it might be impossible to distinguish between the two causes just by history alone. The importance of an accurate diagnosis is, once again, all-important.

However, one medication that would have a logical role in the treatment of genuine stress urinary incontinence is estrogen. As mentioned before, estrogen is necessary for normal urethral coaptation (high pressure in the urethra, resulting from the walls pressing together). A lack of estrogen can sometimes be helpful in the treatment of stress incontinence, but is obviously more applicable in the post-menopausal, older patient. Unfortunately, my experience with estrogen as a treatment for urinary incontinence has been quite disappointing.

There are other medications that have an effect on the urethral sphincter, leading to stronger contractions. Some common cold medications contain ingredients that have this effect. But I doubt if many women have found that their incontinence was improved by such medications when their cold was accompanied by excessive sneezing.

There are two anatomical sites that are targets for drug effects. These are the bladder and also the urethra. The targets for drugs are mainly smooth muscles that are not under conscious control. In the bladder, this is the smooth muscle of the bladder wall, called the detrusor muscle. The urethra has its internal sphincter that can often be manipulated by medication.

Muscles can be in either a contracted or relaxed state. Different effects can be obtained by increasing the relative state of relaxation, or the power of contraction of one of these particular muscles.

For overactive bladder with urgency incontinence, the idea is to prevent abnormal and untimely bladder (detrusor) contractions. For stress urinary incontinence, increasing the tone or strength of the urethral sphincter will be beneficial. For urinary obstruction related to a flaccid bladder muscle, increasing the strength of detrusor contractions will be effective, whereas decreasing the tone of the urethral sphincter will be the goal.

There are different medications that can accomplish one or more of the above effects. Anticholinergic medications have already been mentioned, and are used for detrusor instability and urge incontinence. Examples of these medications include: tolterodine (Detrol® or Unidet® [also named Detrol LA®]), oxybutynin (Ditropan® or Ditropan XL®), flavoxate (Urispas®), and a few others. Some medications can have the effect of relaxing the detrusor muscle while at the same time increasing the strength of the urethra, a very useful combination. Common examples of this are tricyclic antidepressant medications, for instance imipramine (Tofranil), nortriptyline, and doxepin.

Examples of medications that might increase urethral tone are phenylephrine, phenylpropanolamine, and pseudoephedrine.

These medications are common in many common cold medications. While thought to be useful for stress urinary incontinence, I personally have not found them to be very helpful.

Note that none of the above medications are without problems. There are numerous, possibly serious side effects that could occur, and extremely serious drug interactions are possible if combined with various other commonly used medications. For elderly patients who are taking numerous drugs, this is an especially relevant concern. The specifics of these drugs and their interactions are outside the scope of this book. The important thing is to make sure that your physician and pharmacist has a compete list of all medications you are taking. Please take your drug list with you! Some patients have waited five or six months to see me, and then they arrive with no knowledge or information about what medications they are on. Patients could save their physicians a little bit of frustration by taking a list, or the actual medications (*all* of them), to their appointments.

The other side of the medicine coin involves the long list of medications that could interfere with normal urinary function and even cause incontinence or urinary obstruction. Again, this is outside the scope of this text, especially since this list is growing as new medications come on the market. Again, when seeking treatment for urinary dysfunction, it is important that your physician knows exactly what medications you are taking. Today, it is becoming significantly more complicated as a result of increasing herbal and alternative medicinal usage. Very few Western medical practitioners are able to stay up to date with the contents of alternative medicines. They may not be sufficiently aware of potential side effects or drug interactions of common over-the-counter medicinal supplements and alternatives. I find this issue very complicated and I have yet to find a user-friendly, trustworthy, and authoritative source of information that could help. Complicating this is the fact that many of these products are insufficiently labeled, manufactured with poor quality control, and are unregulated.

Pelvic Floor Exercises

As a general rule, the simplest solution likely to succeed should be tried first. One of the first options includes ways to strengthen the pelvic floor muscles. Most women are vaguely aware of the pelvic floor muscle exercises called "Kegels." These exercises involve the repetitive contraction of the levator ani and sphincter muscles to the point of exhaustion. One might see this as "bodybuilding" of the pelvis. Just as bodybuilding is extremely hard work and has to be done diligently and for a long period of time to see any effects, pelvic floor exercises do not provide a quick fix. The television advertisers who promise a miraculously toned body with minimal effort are, without a doubt, lying to you. The same is true regarding Kegels. No matter how many years you've done them; if they are not done regularly and with enough intensity, forget it. It has been my experience that few women obtain good results from exercises alone. Just as most new gym members exercise enthusiastically for three weeks to one month, after which their workouts become progressively more infrequent until they finally stop, so most women stop doing the pelvic exercises, or they do not do them frequently or intensely enough to be of much benefit.

For the highly motivated woman, especially those without severe pelvic fascia or nerve injuries, diligently performed pelvic floor exercises could make a big difference, one that may even lead to a cure. Exercise will increase muscle strength, but unfortunately it has no effect on damaged nerves or fascia, especially tears or disruption. In the presence of significant denervation of the pelvic floor muscles, or obvious fascial detachment, one should have guarded optimism, and indeed studies have found that in such women the results are not as good. However, since it is completely safe and has no negative side effects, everybody should at least consider these exercises as a primary, or at least a complementary, treatment option. To keep motivation high and to be sure that the exercises are done correctly, biofeedback or other professional help is preferable. To get back to the gym analogy, there is a world of difference in results between those who train on their own and those who have a personal trainer. But often this is logistically or financially out of reach for most women.

The following is a very simple and easy-to-understand Kegel exercise program. I found this description of pelvic floor exercises while browsing the Internet. I thought it was an excellent, beautifully descriptive explanation, and would like to share it with a wider audience. Unfortunately I have no idea who the original author is, so I cannot give due credit to the following advice.

For many years, patients have been advised that the proper way to perform Kegel exercises was to activate those pelvic floor muscles that would allow the patient to stop and then start the urinary stream. A better way of describing the proper way to perform Kegel exercises is:

> Imagine that, rather abruptly, you are experiencing a strong need to either pass gas or have a bowel movement; however, the restroom is occupied and you will have to wait a few minutes. What do you do to avoid an accidental stool loss? As you tighten the muscles in your pelvic diaphragm that will prevent that loss of gas/stool, and hold it, imagine that NOW you perceive a strong desire to void urine—but the restroom is STILL occupied! You now have to hold tight both these muscle groups (stool and urine). Do this for 10 seconds. Then relax for 10 seconds. Repeat 10 times in a row (rectal then vaginal). This is called a set. Perform three sets a day for at least six weeks. Properly and diligently performed, there are some studies indicating significant reduction in the need for surgery for stress incontinence after six weeks.

The beauty of Kegel exercises is that there is no need for special equipment, there are no training fees, and you can do them anywhere. Sometimes, patients may not know how to activate these unused muscles, so during a pelvic exam, your doctor can help focus you on the muscles needed during that examination by asking you to tighten here (rectally) and then here (vaginally). By identifying the muscle groups in this way, the proper neuromuscular connections can be made very quickly. Kegel exercises *are* worthwhile if done correctly and consistently.

Consider also that a recent research study from Australia found that tensioning the internal oblique (IO) and the transverses abdominus (TA) muscles during pelvic floor exercises is of cardinal importance to generate adequately strong contractions in the pelvic floor muscles. It was found to be impossible to generate strong pelvic floor contractions without also recruiting these abdominal muscles. Identifying these particular muscles to preferentially contract them is not intuitive, and this is another reason to get physiotherapy.

To strengthen any muscle, the exercises have to attain maximal muscle contraction, thereby leading to exhaustion of the muscle. Only in doing that, will the muscle adapt by getting stronger—

instant evolution on a small scale! Previous instruction that encouraged keeping the abdominals totally relaxed might not have been the best advice. Just strengthening the abdominals per se might contribute to pelvic floor health.

Vaginal Cones

Vaginal cones are cone-shaped weights that are used, in effect, to do vaginal weight training. Progressively heavier weights are placed in the vagina and the patient tries to keep them in for as long as possible by tightening the vaginal and, by implication, the pelvic floor muscles. In some ways, it is easier to use the cones than to perform Kegels. The vagina senses that the cone is slipping, and that almost subconsciously leads to contractions of the pelvic floor muscles. I have had some success with cones in my own practice. The most poignant illustration of their success is a testimonial from a very happy patient. She told me that when she "graduated" from using the heaviest (also slimmest) cone, she took her husband for a second honeymoon. From the twinkle in her eyes, I believe they had a heck of a good time!

Electrical and Electromagnetic Muscle Stimulation

Many people are familiar with the electrical muscle stimulation process used by physiotherapists. This modality is ordinarily used for rehabilitation after injuries as an adjunct to the overall therapy plan. Similar equipment can be utilized to stimulate the levator ani muscles. It is not a popular method (for obvious reasons), but like almost everything, it has its enthusiasts. Recent studies maintain that magnetic stimulation has demonstrated success in the treatment of bladder (detrusor) instability and urge incontinence. New research is looking into electromagnetic stimulation of pelvic muscles, something that is outside the scope of this book.

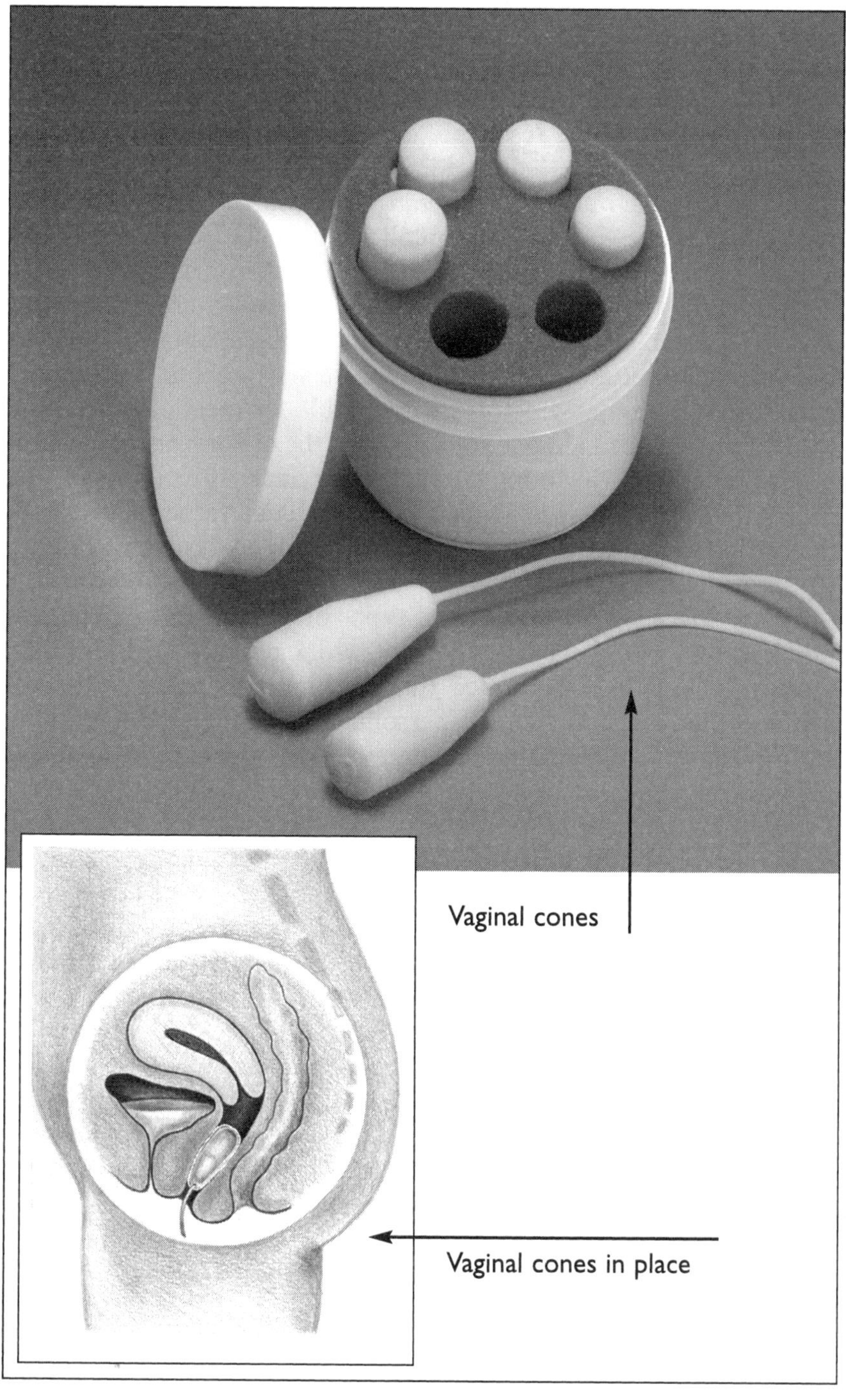
Vaginal cones
Vaginal cones in place

Pessaries

No discussion regarding urinary incontinence and prolapse would be complete without a section on pessaries. This involves the wearing of a device in the vagina that effectively supports and pushes the bladder neck area upward. Although it works effectively for some, I have found the acceptability level to be low over the long term, especially in younger women. This is not surprising. Pessaries are sometimes uncomfortable, need to be cleaned periodically, and usually need to be removed prior to intercourse. Finally, and perhaps most importantly, they do not cure the problem but merely mask the symptoms, which is unacceptable for most patients. As a result, they are used almost exclusively in the old or frail, or for temporary relief while awaiting surgery. They have a much bigger role in patients with prolapse as their main problem, rather than incontinence. Many research studies confirm the low success rates with pessaries for incontinence.

Since there are many different types of pessaries available, it is quite an art to find the one that will work best for an individual woman. I have been informed that my limited success with pessaries is the result of my own personal counseling strategies, possibly because I am, by nature, a surgeon. Although I do believe that I have been trying my best to be objective when counseling patients, I accept the inevitability of some truth to the allegation. If someone goes to a physiotherapist for counseling, physiotherapy is likely going to be found as the best option. When going to a dedicated pessary clinic, the same would be found. I believe the only way around this dilemma would be an integrated, multimodality pelvic floor clinic. Only in this way will personal biases be minimized.

One last word on pessaries: There is a relatively simple way to find out whether a pessary might help. Using one or two (depending on vaginal size) tampons has a similar, although lesser, effect than a specifically designed pessary. Many women are very hesitant about the "foreign object" nature of a pessary, but are quite used to inserting a tampon. If a tampon diminishes the stress incontinence, it is likely that a pessary will help even more. In these situations surgery is also very likely to be effective (oops . . . that bias again).

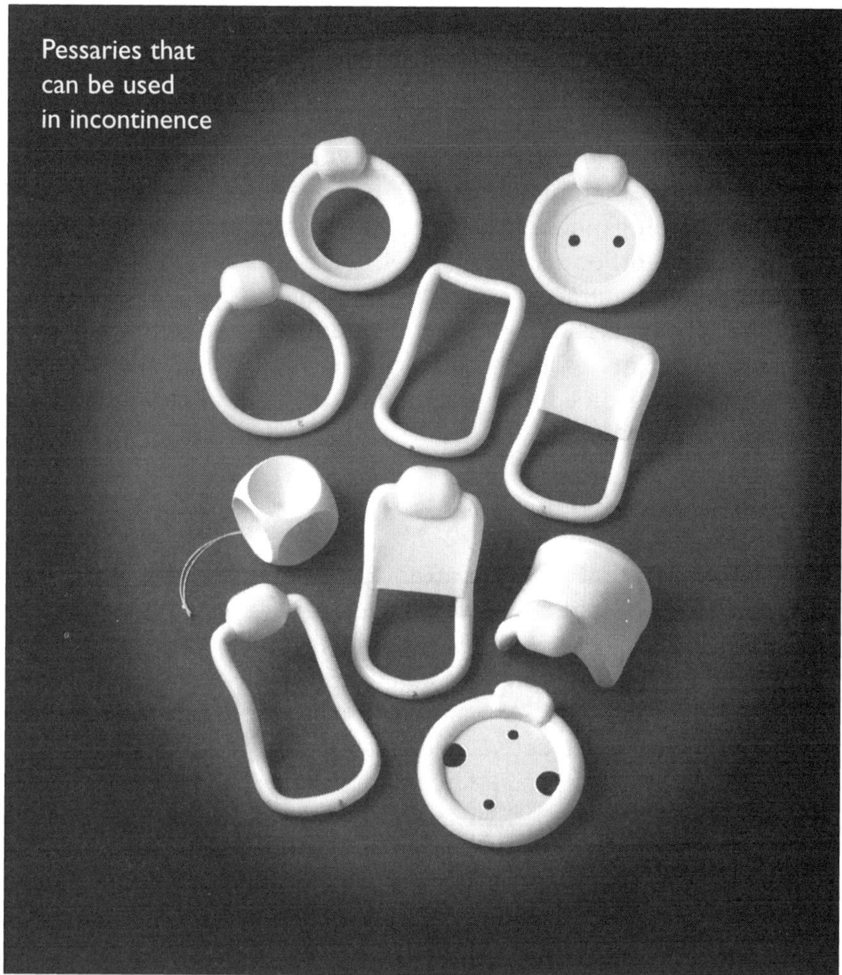
Pessaries that can be used in incontinence

Urethral Plugs

One further nonsurgical management option for stress urinary incontinence is urethral plugs or inserts. There are various different kinds of these devices, and I will not try to describe them in any detail. These devices generally work by applying them to the urethral meatus (opening of the urethra), and physically obstructing the flow of urine. Basically, some of the earlier devices were simply plugs, whereas the more commonly used ones today almost look like soft silicone catheters, without a canal. The device is placed through the urethra, and has an expanding balloonlike bulb on the end that is inside the bladder, thereby obstructing the flow of urine through the urethra.

These devices are single-use only and are usually used during a particular activity. For instance, the device might be inserted just prior to playing a tennis match, and removed afterward. Problems with urethral plugs include a higher rate of urinary tract infections and the discomfort of inserting something through the urethra. As a result of low patient acceptance, many of these devices have come and gone. My experience with them is minimal, and that holds true for many other gynecologists or urogynecologists. However, they may very well become more accepted and popular in the future.

PHYSIOTHERAPY

It is well known that a large percentage of women with stress urinary incontinence can benefit from pelvic floor strengthening via biofeedback. One of the best ways to accomplish pelvic strengthening is under the direct supervision of physiotherapists with a special interest in this field. As said earlier, having a personal trainer could be the difference between success and disillusionment.

Physiotherapists specializing in this field will not only teach patients how to contract their pelvic floor muscles, but will guide them step-by-step to develop core abdominal strength and teach them how to prevent episodes of stress incontinence through anticipatory tightening of the pelvic floor muscles. Although it seems that tightening the levator muscles (pelvic floor muscles) should be a simple task to learn, this is simply not the case.

Many physiotherapists also have the training and equipment to do electromyography testing on the pelvic floor muscles to determine whether they are innervated or not. This testing determines whether the muscles have an intact and functioning nerve supply. Without this, muscles cannot function, and any attempt at pelvic floor strengthening by any method would be an absolute waste of time and money.

In Canada and many other countries, this kind of physiotherapy is usually not covered by government-run public health insurance plans. This obviously will weigh heavily in the decision making of individual women. In my practice, I have found the cost issue to be a significant negative. Many women in the Canadian provinces where I have practiced do not have extended health care coverage, and thus have no insurance for physiotherapy. This then becomes an out-of-pocket expense. Although there are many patients who simply cannot afford the additional expense, there is also the issue of expectations. In Canada, as in many other countries with socialist medical systems, patients' expectations of free medical care for everything become a significant deterrent to purchasing additional care which might be helpful but not lifesaving. As a result, this kind of physiotherapy may be extremely underutilized in many countries.

In the U.S., each private health plan will have different rules as to whether physiotherapy is covered or not. Recently, Medicare adopted coverage of biofeedback treatment for patients who have failed a documented trial of pelvic muscle exercise (PME) training.

Behavioral Modification

I'm often amazed to hear how much water patients consume. Some people apparently have the belief that they *have* to drink a certain amount of water per day—often an inordinate number of glasses that they religiously hold to. It becomes an obsession! There is *no* such absolute rule! Of course it's not healthy to be dehydrated, but to think you have to drink a certain number of glasses of water per day is incorrect. Just decreasing their fluid intake, and being careful about *when* they drink and *what* they drink *when*, has improved the incontinence problems of many people.

Here are a few commonsense tips:

- Don't consume more fluids than necessary. Only drink when thirsty.
- Don't drink before bedtime (about two hours before).
- Decrease or eliminate caffeine (coffee, ordinary tea). Caffeine is one of the strongest bladder irritants out there.
- Double voiding sometimes helps. Empty your bladder and then go again immediately. This can help since the bladder may not empty completely the first time.

- If you're having problems with incontinence during sexual intercourse, empty your bladder before having sex.
- Keep a voiding diary. You can obtain one from your doctor or one can be found at www.depend.com.

Voiding diaries work by showing the association between activities, fluid intake, and episodes of urinary incontinence. This newly found knowledge often enables patients to modify or time their fluid intake in relation to certain activities that they plan for the day.

NINE
Surgery for Treating Urinary Incontinence

AN OPEN LETTER

After a prolonged labor and a difficult forceps delivery, I was left with a weakened pelvic floor. As a busy mom working full time, I found the increasing necessity of wearing some form of feminine protection a chore. Seventeen years later, I had a vaginal hysterectomy and repair that lasted for more than three years, but gradually incontinence returned and I resorted to wearing some sort of protection again. In 1994, I underwent surgery known as the Pereya Needle Suspension. It was not successful. I thought I was doomed to frequent visits to the bathroom and constant use of incontinence products. Two months later, I heard about a surgery called TVT Tension-Free Support. I was referred to a surgeon, and because of the two previous surgeries, it was suggested that I undergo urodynamic and cyctoscopy testing first. Results from those tests indicated that I could have the TVT surgery. I have been pleased with the results. It has greatly improved my ability to stay continent, but Kegel exercises do play a continued part in strengthening my pelvic floor muscles. With newer surgical techniques being studied and used, and appropriate preoperative assessments being done, gynecologists can offer simple and effective surgeries to many women suffering from incontinence.

Claire, a registered nurse

Thoughts on Surgery

Some studies tout the success of behavioral modification or other conservative treatments for urinary incontinence. These studies often employ the term "statistical significance," meaning that effectiveness is measured in decreased incontinence episodes for a specific time period. This is all great, and I'm certainly not disputing the fact that conservative management options have a large role to play, and in many cases should be utilized first. However, I don't think that women should be satisfied with merely decreasing their incontinence episodes by one or two per day. With the minimal invasiveness of some of today's surgical procedures, as well as the very high likelihood of a complete cure, I believe it is a disservice to women to keep them from the knowledge and access to certain surgical procedures. They can make an informed decision whether they wish to continue conservative treatment options or consider surgery.

It is not for me to decide if a reduction in symptoms from conservative management techniques is a success, and that they should disqualify a woman from a surgery that may cure her completely. Yes, it might be "success" on paper, but for certain women even one leak at the wrong time might be devastating.

This should not be seen as discrediting conservative management of urinary incontinence. Other than time and monetary commitments, it is risk free, which cannot be said of surgery, however minimally invasive. But I do not think withholding a surgical option as a result of an arbitrary "improvement" is ethical either. Today's new surgical procedures have so many advantages over those of years past, that not informing the patient of their existence is, in my view, unethical.

No Ideal Surgical Solution

Consider the following:

> The advance of science can be measured by the rate at which exceptions to previously held laws accumulate. The corollaries: (1) Exceptions always outnumber the rules. (2) There are always exceptions to established exceptions. (3) By the time one masters the exceptions, no one recalls the rules to which they apply.[1]

It is a well-known surgical principal that the more surgical procedures there are for the same problem, the more likely it is that none of the procedures are ideal. The reason for this is obvious. If there were one perfect surgical solution, everybody would be doing the same thing. Urinary incontinence and, specifically, stress urinary incontinence, is one of those areas where there are an incredible number of different surgical procedures performed. The gynecological and urological literature is full of contradictory and speculative opinions, which makes the evaluation and comparison of the different surgical procedures very difficult. One insightful commentator once stated that urogynecology is that field with one test and a hundred operations. This was not intended as a compliment. Fortunately, the specialty has progressed, although not far enough.

Obstacles in Research

One of the main problems, in terms of comparing different studies, is the fact that there is no uniform outcome measurement used by researchers. As such, it is poignant to consider the whole picture principle:

> Research scientists are so wrapped up in their own narrow endeavors that they cannot possibly see the whole picture of anything, including their own research.[2]

The problem is that different definitions are used, not only for the initial problem but also for the outcome results. Some studies use subjective measurements (surveys filled in by patients) to determine surgical results, whereas others use objective (urodynamic testing, like the cystometrogram) studies. Some of the newer surgical procedures and the follow-up periods after a surgery vary widely, too. For example, laparoscopic and newer sling procedures have relatively short follow-up periods. This causes uncertainty about the long-term results. Certain new procedures, and even certain synthetic and animal tissues that are used during some of these surgeries, do not have to go through strict trials, since showing that one is substantially similar to something else already on the market exempts it from going through its own trials. While there are obvious risks and problems involved with this approach, this has allowed for speedy implementation of new ideas that might be evolutionary, if not revolutionary.

Additionally, the fragmentation of research is compounded by a certain amount of rivalry between urological and gynecological colleagues, leading each specialty to carry out research in isolation, with little sharing of information. I have been quite shocked by the apparent intensity that this rivalry sometimes achieves. By now one would think that the different specialties have developed enough self-confidence to not feel threatened by other specialties that might overlap their narrowly defined field of interest. Unfortunately, this is not the case. Between urogynecology and urology, the historical relationship has been one of confrontation, as well as a certain mutual disdain, rather than cooperation. In my opinion, this is very unfortunate since each specialty has so much to give, and the two are ideally suited to complement one another for the betterment of patient care.

Expected Cure Rates

Objective cure rates for various surgical procedures vary widely. Realistically, the most that could be expected after the primary surgery (first operation for the problem) with the most appropriate procedure would be cure rates of approximately 75 to 85 percent after about five years. There is a definite element of time decay with most procedures (more recurrent problems as time goes on), which tends to be significantly more pronounced in patients with medical conditions such as obesity and chronic cough from smoking and asthma. The genetically determined strength of the body's connective tissue is an important factor not only for the immediate operative result, but also for the likelihood of a relapse. General lifestyle issues (heavy lifting, etc.) also play a role in the possibility or probability of recurrence of the problem. The expectation should not necessarily be for recurrence however, since for many women the cure lasts a lifetime. But there are no guarantees. Patients can help to make lifetime cure more likely by following the lifestyle advice given, and by making a lifelong habit of thinking of pelvic floor health. Just as general fitness is exceptionally important for overall quality of life, pelvic floor fitness is also important for optimum functioning and prevention of the problems—and prevention of recurrences.

It is important to note that often, anti-incontinence surgery has to be combined with additional procedures. Most common are those associated with the correction of pelvic organ prolapse. These are often vaginal repairs of cystocele, rectocele, enterocele, and/or uterine prolapse or vaginal vault prolapse. Hysterectomy is often done concurrently. Many of these vaginal reconstructive surgical procedures will determine the appropriateness of certain anticontinence procedures.

Vaginal Surgery

The original surgery performed for urinary incontinence was the anterior vaginal repair. This procedure is done entirely via the vagina and is still performed routinely for the repair of a cystocele (prolapse of the anterior vaginal wall, leading to a "fallen bladder"). Basically, the cystocele is repaired, and one or more extra sutures are placed in the fascia underneath the bladder neck to pull the bladder neck up. Deep bites are taken into this fascia, which are then pulled together. This procedure was originally described by Howard A. Kelly and is sometimes still called the "Kelly plication." The problem is that the sutures are not fixed to any strong anchor points but only to the fascia itself. Since failure of this same fascia probably contributed to the original problem, and since resorbable sutures are used, it is no surprise that this surgical procedure is the least effective over the

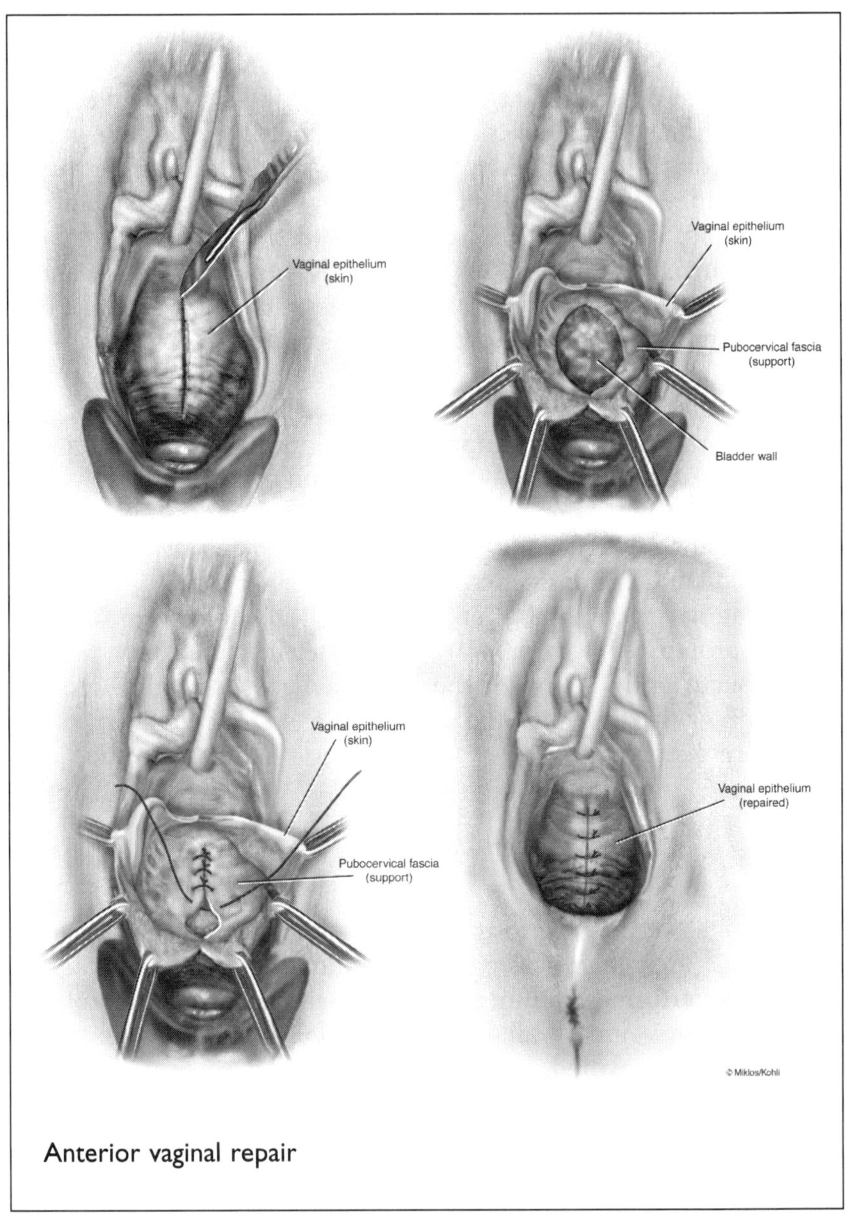

Anterior vaginal repair

long term. Because fascia that has pulled away from the pelvic side-walls (called "paravaginal defects") is the most common cause of anterior descent in the first place, it is almost ridiculous to imagine that bundling it up in the midline (which is what is done during standard interior repair) will create long-term support. So a cystocele and concomitant stress incontinence often recur if treated this way, even when the surgery is performed perfectly.

Abdominal Procedures

The more appropriate surgery for genuine stress incontinence anchors the pelvic fascia to a strong point that is higher than the urethra, effectively suspending urethral support as well as lifting it up to a more normal position. Surgeries that fall into this category include the Marshall-Marchetti-Krantz procedure, the Burch procedure, certain sling procedures, and various needle suspension operations. I will not discuss these operations in detail but will point out a few important factors.

The Marshall-Marchetti-Krantz procedure (usually called the Marshall-Marchetti or the MMK procedure) was the original procedure described in 1949 by V. F. Marshall, A. A. Marchetti, and K. E. Krantz. It uses the pelvic bone periostium (bone lining) as its strong anchor point.

The Burch procedure uses a ligament on top of the pubic bone as its anchor point. It has become the more accepted procedure because of certain theoretical advantages over the Marshall-Marchetti procedure. These include less risk of obstruction of the urethra, and the absence of the risk of osteitis (inflammation or infection) of the pubic bone. Both of these operations are usually done as abdominal procedures and so carry many of the implications of abdominal surgery.

Another surgical procedure that has gained quite a following over the last few years is paravaginal repair. This surgery makes a lot of intuitive sense, since its whole premise is the repair of the causal abnormality by reattachment of the pelvic fascia to the pelvic sidewall. This part of the pelvic fascia is the pubocervical fascia, the most important part of the vaginal fascia involved in the support of the anterior vaginal wall and therefore closely related to the urethra. The premise of paravaginal repair is that many cases of genuine stress urinary incontinence, especially in the setting of a cystocele, happen when the pubocervical fascia tears away from the lateral pelvic sidewalls where it is attached to the so-called white line of the pelvis (the medical term is the "arcus tendineus fascia pelvis"). If

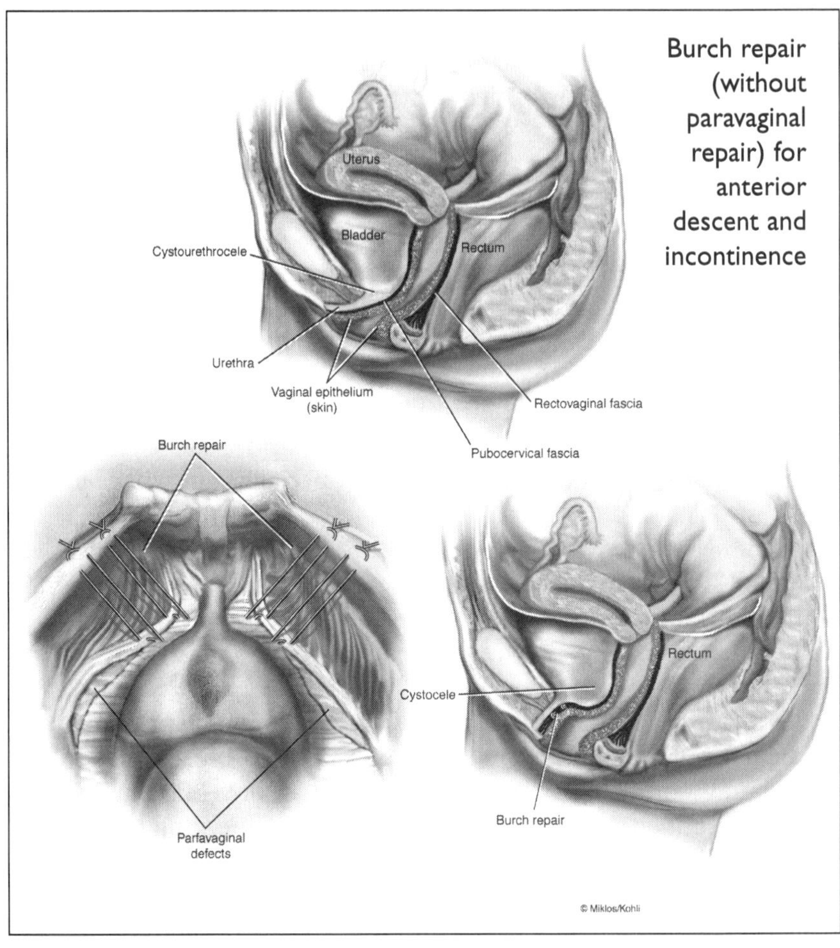

Burch repair (without paravaginal repair) for anterior descent and incontinence

you think back to our pelvic trampoline model, this attachment of the fascia to the pelvic sidewalls corresponds to the rolled up edges of the white sheet that were attached, not to the frame itself, but to the underlying canvas that represents the levator ani muscle group. This thickening of fascia forms the white line (arcus tendineus).

A rupture leading to prolapse and possibly incontinence can occur on the left or the right side, but has interestingly been found to be somewhat more common on the right. Reattachment of this fascia can be accomplished during a Burch or a Marshall-Marchetti procedure by adding certain steps to the procedure. Unfortunately, too many surgeons (urologists and gynecologists alike) totally ignore rupture as an underlying cause for many cases of cystocele

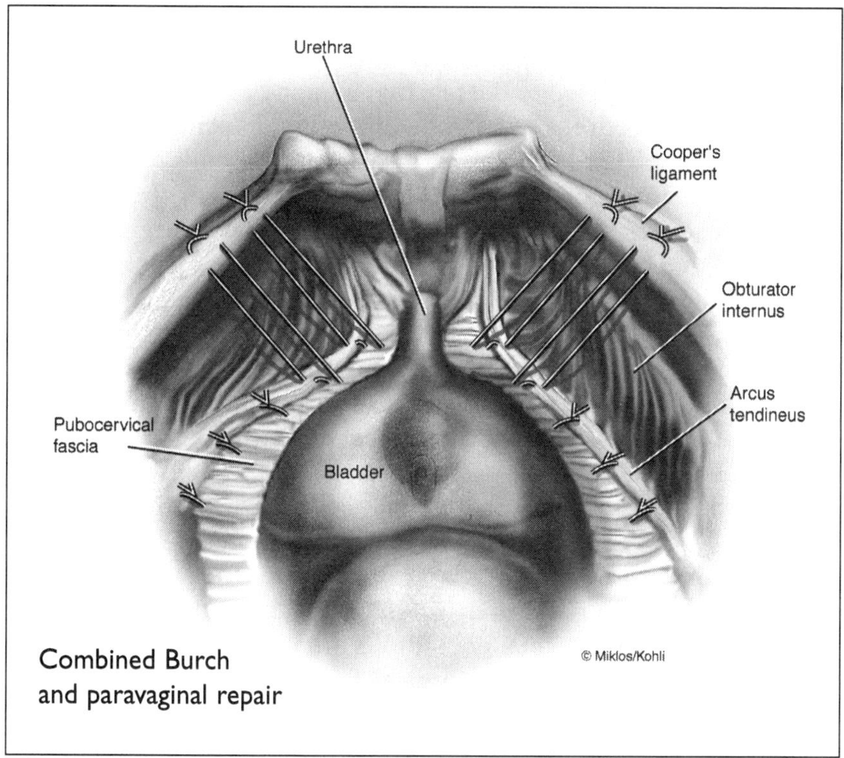

Combined Burch and paravaginal repair

and urinary incontinence. I believe this results from their incomplete understanding of the pelvic fascia and its disorders. They fail to seek the underlying problem, and therefore they are unaware of what should be done to correct it. They resort instead to a one-shoe-fits-all approach, and perform the same surgery on everybody. In my opinion, this is a dubious approach with poor long-term results.

Paravaginal repair has also been described as a vaginal procedure, but unfortunately this is far more difficult and certainly not part of the average gynecologists' surgery options. Laparoscopic paravaginal repair is better accomplished.

Laparoscopic Surgery

Surgeons are now able to perform certain procedures laparoscopically (minimal access surgery or "keyhole" surgery). Although it seems as if the end result is comparable to open surgery, its success is still controversial. Some studies have found that the laparoscopic Burch procedure has poorer success than open Burch. Many experts feel this could be related to the fact that in many of these studies, the laparoscopic procedures were done differently in principle than the open procedures. For instance, whereas most surgeons would place at least two sutures on each side of the bladder neck during open Burch procedures, in many of these laparoscopic procedures only one was placed on each side. Others utilized various techniques that supposedly made the procedure quicker and faster. Of course, most of those modifications were made due to the inherent technical difficulties of the laparoscopic procedure. In the end, apples were compared to oranges. The procedures are simply not the same. Many experts feel that in similarly performed procedures, with only the access being different, the results should be exactly the same. Although this makes good common sense, I think the verdict is still out. Today, commonly performed laparoscopic surgeries for incontinence and prolapse are laparoscopic Burch procedures *combined with* paravaginal repair. The Burch is done first, and the paravaginal repair subsequently. Permanent sutures are used. The sutures often are placed through the pubocervical fascia and through the full thickness of the vaginal wall, often right into the vagina. Usually the sutures become covered with vaginal epithelium (vaginal skin), but occasionally I've had to remove a stitch from the vagina—an event that should not be cause for significant concern.

There are two possible ways to approach the laparoscopic paravaginal repair or Burch—either through the extraperitoneal or transperitoneal approach. I will briefly describe the difference since this will almost certainly come up in any discussion a patient might have preoperatively.

TRANSPERITONEAL

A thin membrane of tissue lines the body cavities. In the abdominal cavity this membrane is called the "peritoneum." The flimsiness of this layer belies its importance to our health. Breaching this layer during surgery, for instance, creates the possibility of adhesions, intra-abdominal infections, etc. During transperitoneal laparoscopic procedures, the instruments are placed through the peritoneum, and

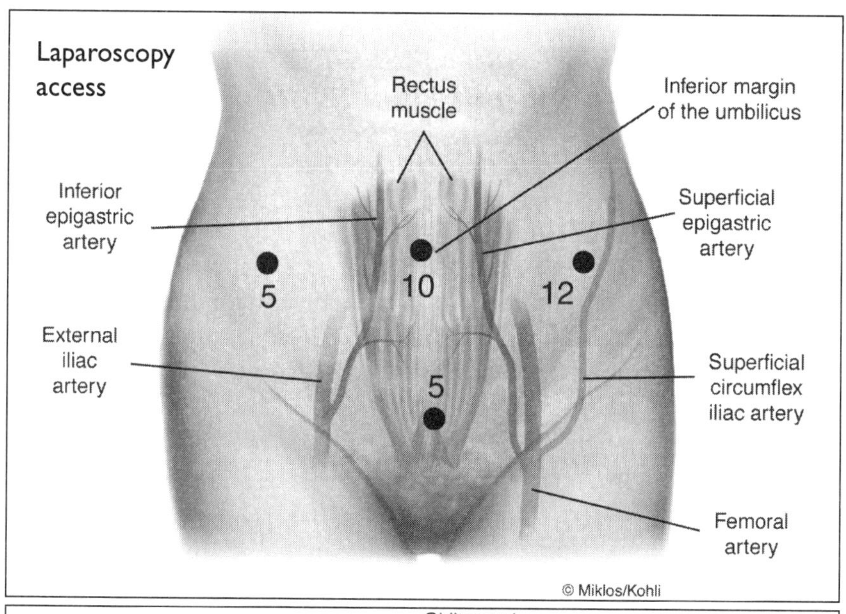
Laparoscopy access
Rectus muscle
Inferior margin of the umbilicus
Inferior epigastric artery
Superficial epigastric artery
5
10
12
External iliac artery
5
Superficial circumflex iliac artery
Femoral artery
© Miklos/Kohli

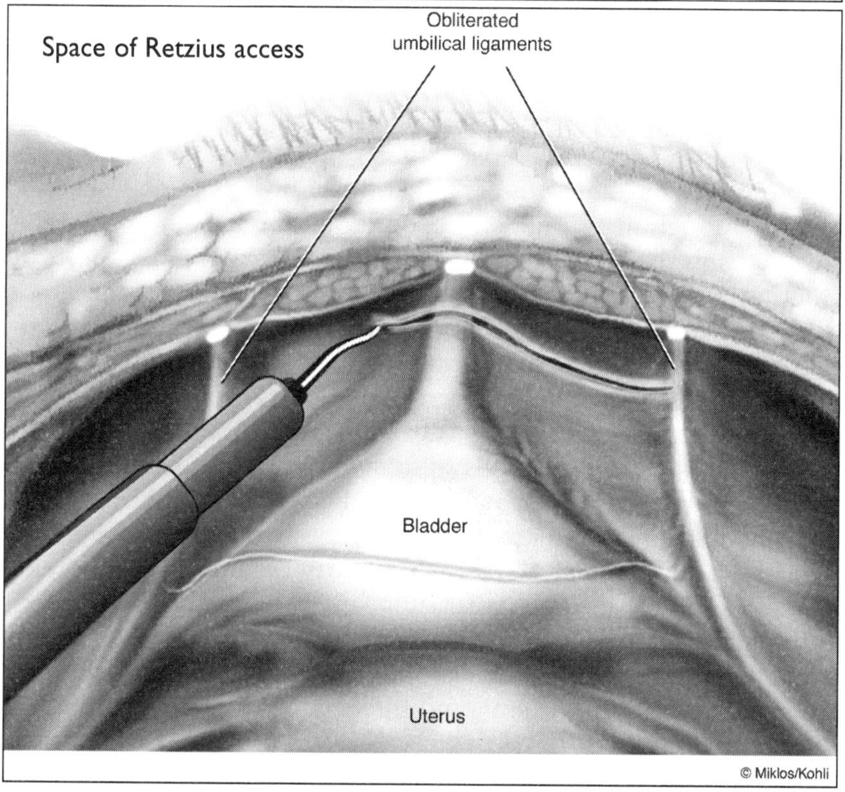

Space of Retzius access
Obliterated umbilical ligaments
Bladder
Uterus
© Miklos/Kohli

thus one is working inside the body cavity. This approach is the one used when other procedures need to be done at the same time, for instance treatment of endometriosis or suspension operations for the uterus or vaginal vault.

To reach the area where the bladder neck sutures are placed for the Burch procedure, one has to dissect between the peritoneal lining and bladder, to gain access to the space of Retzius (see illustration on page 97). This is the potential space above the pubocervical fascia where all abdominal anti-incontinence procedures are performed. This is more difficult than it sounds, and there is some risk of entering the bladder during the dissection.

EXTRAPERITONEAL

The extraperitoneal approach is ideal when the anti-incontinence procedure is the only procedure planned. It is performed by sliding a deflated balloon from the umbilicus (belly button) underneath the skin down to behind the pubic bone, staying above the peritoneum, between the peritoneum and the posterior sheath of the rectus abdominal muscles. The balloon then is inflated, and in the process opens up the space of Retzius. All instruments inserted only penetrate through the skin, muscle fascia (including the rectus sheath), but *not* through the peritoneum. The procedure is quick, opens the space effectively, and does not have the negative potential effects of entering the abdominal cavity. One of the common effects of extraperitoneal laparoscopy is "surgical emphysema." After the procedure, patients may have gas bubbles under their skin, sometimes over a very wide area of their body. Although anesthetists are usually none too happy about it if not forewarned (there is a concern that it may interfere with breathing as a result of pressure in the neck), it is almost always innocuous and goes away rapidly.

It stands to reason that with this approach, other procedures for which intra-abdominal access is necessary cannot be performed. However, this is an ideal access for laparoscopic Burch and paravaginal repair procedures. Unfortunately, it cannot be used in patients who have had previous abdominal surgery, since the tissues are stuck together in the scar, and the dissection balloon cannot be slid into place.

The immediate postoperative recovery after laparoscopic procedures is certainly easier and quicker than for open procedures, with discharge often on the same or the next day, but patients still have to take the same precautions for the first six weeks to three months. These include a ban on anything that would put a strain on the sutures like lifting, straining, repetitive bending, or sexual activity. Before the healing process has had a chance to form strong attachments to keep the bladder and urethra in position, the newly suspended fascia only hangs from a few sutures, which could easily come undone. The real recovery period is thus, in my view, often simplistically minimized. A good rule of thumb for postoperative activity after surgery for urinary incontinence or pelvic organ prolapse is:

First six weeks: NO lifting. NO sex. Walking, swimming, stationary biking is OK. Prevent constipation.

Second six weeks: Light lifting only. Sex OK. More intense exercise OK but nothing putting undue strain on pelvic floor like jumping, high-impact aerobics, weight lifting in erect position (like squatting). Light weights in nonerect position, for instance dumbbell flies when lying on the back is acceptable. I'm often asked about golf, which is probably OK to play one round of golf after six weeks to two months, provided you don't try to hit the green in one on a par-five hole. Use higher number clubs and swing easily. Ride a cart. *Do not carry your golf bag!* Enjoy your outing, and if it is any time between November and May: think of me, who will still be freezing in the Canadian prairies.

Another problem with laparoscopic surgery is the significantly increased operating time it takes to perform these procedures. This factor has led many (if not most) gynecologists, who started off enthusiastically on the laparoscopic bandwagon, to abandon it after a while. This especially becomes a problem in countries like Canada where operating room time is in very short supply, and where surgeons get paid a flat (government set) fee for a procedure, whichever way it is performed. Most surgeons have realized that with the time it takes, and with their available operating room time, they cannot afford to do it. The minimal fee paid for many procedures in Canada has had the unfortunate but predictable effect of focusing the minds of surgeons on volume, rather than quality. The surgeon's fee for some procedures in the United States can be up to ten times that what surgeons in Canada get paid for exactly the same procedure. This is without taking currency exchange rates into consideration. A Canadian gynecologist might thus be much more reluctant to learn to perform procedures that will take much longer, even if they are ultimately better for patients.

A few gynecologists I know have become extremely proficient at performing open Burch procedures through a very tiny incision. Besides requiring less operating time, the procedure still provides most of the benefits of laparoscopic surgery, such as early discharge.

Needle Procedures

Needle suspension operations are mostly done from the vaginal side, with only one or two small abdominal incisions (approximately one-half to three-quarters of an inch each). The endopelvic fascia on each side of the bladder neck is sutured, and the sutures are pulled past the bladder, behind the pubic bone, and through the abdominal wall using a long needle (hence the name). They are then tied in such a way that they are suspended from the rectus sheath. Although very effective over the short term in the right patient, the drawback is that the anchor point used is usually the rectus sheath, and it is not strong enough over the long term to prevent a repeat prolapse. The rectus sheath is a relatively thick fascia layer covering the two big abdominal muscles called the "rectus muscles." Since this fascia is understandably weaker than ligament or bone, the sutures may cut through or tear out. As a result, these operations are usually performed in the less active and older patients who might be anesthetic risks for larger abdominal procedures. There are numerous examples of different modifications of this operation, some attaching the sutures to the Cooper's ligaments, the same ligaments where the Burch suspension sutures are attached (see illustration on page 95). This is however a difficult thing to do, and often not successful, even if attempted. Needle suspension surgery has come and gone. Very few people are performing them today. Their long-term success rates are poor. There are much better procedures. If your physician wants to do a needle procedure, get a second opinion.

SLINGS

Sling procedures are a large group of diverse operations. Because there are so many varieties, I will keep my comments general and suggest that you ask any surgeon who suggests a sling operation the following questions:

1. Why a sling in the first place?
2. What material will be used for the sling and why? What is the data—rejection rates, erosion rates, infection rates—for that particular sling material and what is the possibility of transmission of disease?
3. What is the basis of your enthusiasm for the suggested sling material? Is it the one or two cases you have done who have (so far) not had problems? What is the data on the material? Has it been approved for this application?
4. Why do you want to do a specific kind of sling, and what exactly is the long-term outcome data for that specific method? Is it just your personal experimental procedure, or is it a procedure that has been studied and has data behind it?
5. Do you have any conflict of interest regarding the choice of material?

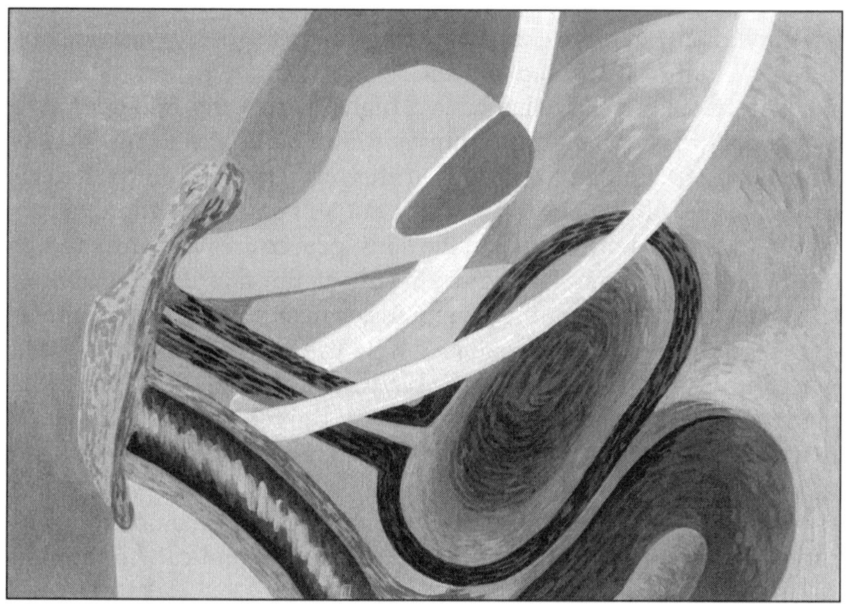

From these questions the reader might infer that I have a certain reservation regarding slings, yet they probably have the best long-term success rates. Why then the above hesitation? Well, the reason goes back to the saying about the one test and the hundred procedures . . . there are *many* kinds of sling procedures. There are slings that use the patient's own abdominal fascia, or muscle from the patient's leg. There are slings utilizing fascia from cadavers (dead bodies), either rectus fascia (abdominal) or fascia lata (leg). There are slings that use fascia from pig's skin, or from the submucosa (internal layer) of the pig's bowel. There are also slings that use vaginal skin as a patch. Then there are the numerous different kinds of synthetic slings. In truth, one can hardly compare one sling to another, as they are so diverse.

Sling procedures incorporate suspension material underneath the bladder neck and urethra, which is then sutured to different anchor points. In addition to the elevation effect (which can also be achieved with Burch procedures), the sling also creates more direct compression of the urethra. Traditionally, these procedures were usually done in patients with dysfunction of the internal urethral continence components, a condition especially common in patients with a history of previous anti-incontinence surgery. This has changed completely to the point where they are often considered appropriate for most patients as primary procedures. Slings have traditionally been more common with urologists than gynecologists, although that has changed as well.

Unfortunately, they also have a higher intra- and postoperative complication rate, including injuries to the bladder and urethra, as well as obstruction and difficulty urinating. The need for catheterization, either indwelling or intermittent self-catheterization, is certainly increased with compressive sling procedures as compared to the Burch procedure. This is the result of the fact that traditional slings are done by elevating the bladder neck with the sling material, regardless of what material was used. The sling had been placed underneath the area of the bladder neck, and an attempt was made to pull the bladder neck up behind the pubic bone. This often led to prolonged obstruction, meaning that patients had significant difficulty with postoperative voiding. If they cannot void sufficiently, patients are subject to prolonged catheterization or self-catheterization to empty their bladders. Intermittent catheterization is the preferred way to manage postincontinence surgery voiding difficulties. It is easily managed by most dexterous and mentally competent patients and it takes only a few minutes to empty the bladder. This will allow women to go home while they await the normalization of spontaneous urination.

It is common to continue to have some difficulties with voiding, for instance slow stream, slow start, or the need to push on the lower abdomen to enable complete bladder emptying. Occasionally, release of the sling is required for correction of prolonged obstruction. It is interesting that even if the sling needs to be cut (it is seldom if ever necessary to remove it), the effectiveness of the surgery most commonly remains.

More serious potential problems with slings include rejection or erosion of the sling material. These complications lead to an inflammatory reaction and reappearance of the sling inside the vagina, or more seriously, inside the bladder or urethra. The only treatment that will usually help is removal. These problems, as well as infection of the sling material, have been much more prevalent with certain older sling materials not commonly used anymore. Some of the modern materials utilized have low erosion and rejection rates, and are more resistant to infections.

Bone-Anchoring Procedures

Many other innovative techniques have been developed to affect elevation and suspension of the bladder neck in an effort to cure stress urinary incontinence. After the Achilles' heel of the needle procedures became known, namely that the sutures tear out of their anchoring point (the rectus fascia), techniques were sought to anchor slings to solid structures unlikely to suffer the same fate. One of the ways developed, that is still in use today, is bone-anchoring technique. These are mostly vaginal procedures where ingenious devices are used to effectively put screws into the backside of the pubic bone. The sling material is placed around the urethra at the level of the bladder neck, and after appropriate tension is employed, the sling is screwed to the back of the pubis. The suspension is strong, and the device works (so I've been told, never having used it personally). However, there are a few reasons why it is not very popular: (1) the device is very expensive, and (2) there is a problem of osteitis pubis. This is a condition of inflammation (not infection—this is another possibility altogether) of the pubic bone where the screws enter the bone. It has been found to be a significant problem, not because it is frequent, but because of the severe pain and disability it can cause, if it develops.

TVT: A New Procedure

A new and, in my view, extremely exciting procedure was introduced to North America in 1999. This is the TVT or "Tension-free Vaginal Tape" procedure. The procedure was developed in Upsala, Sweden, by Dr. Ulf Ulmsten, and was clinically tested and introduced in Europe a few years before coming to North America. It evolved from a revolutionary new view of incontinence and urethral support (see discussion of integral theory of urinary continence in chapter 7), placing more emphasis on distal (closer to the exit) urethral fascia support and discounting the elevation aspects of all other incontinence procedures.

It is performed as an outpatient procedure, takes about twenty to twenty-five minutes to do, and involves only a small incision in the vagina under the urethra, and very small abdominal incisions. Different than with most other anti-incontinence procedures where patients might have considerable difficulty with urination after the operation, most (about 90 percent) of TVT patients will void within the first twenty-four hours. For this reason, the TVT operation is the only anti-incontinence operation where a catheter is not usually required, and where patients routinely go home the same day as their anti-incontinence surgery. A further attractive aspect of the procedure is that it can be done under a very light spinal anesthetic or under local anesthetic only. In fact, it is important that the patient be awake and is able to cooperate, since part of the procedure is a dynamic test of leakage, to measure just how tight the TVT tape should be placed. The idea is to create support for the urethra with a synthetic tape, to replace the lost support of the damaged fascia. The tape is placed tension free, but just tight enough to objectively (visibly, by having the patient cough) stop the incontinence. It is placed past the bladder with special needles that then exit the abdominal wall through the small incisions. Here the procedure differs radically from the needle procedures. Whereas the sutures of the needle procedures are sewn across the rectus sheath for their support, with the possible problems of cutting through, the tape of the TVT is left without any need for suturing. Suffice it to say that the tape has been designed in such a way that suturing is unnecessary. Although it sounds incredulous at first, its design concept is really brilliant; and best of all, it works.

Although the TVT procedure has gained international acceptance and the preliminary reports indicate excellent cure rates, it needs to be noted that it is still a relatively new procedure, without very long-term follow-up data available. Nevertheless, the first studies of up to six-year data have now been published and are almost universally excellent.

At the 2001 meeting of the American Urogynecology Society, there were an inordinate number of posters, lectures, and research studies presented on TVT. The data has been so impressive, that even the naysayers are starting to take note. The success of the TVT operation has had the predictable result of creating a flurry of would-be innovators of competing systems. Recently, a similar procedure was promoted as a supposedly safer one since it is done from the abdominal side in a way that is similar to earlier needle procedures. The theoretical benefits include the possibility of a reduction of serious complications. A similar tape is used for TVT.

Interestingly, I feel that the copying of the basic philosophy and mechanism of TVT shows vindication and acceptance of the tension-free concept as a significant evolution in our understanding of urinary incontinence in women.

I have been doing TVTs since 1999 and it has revolutionized my practice. I cannot imagine practicing without the ability to do this one procedure. Yet it is still surgery. There have been reports of a few very serious complications, and even a few deaths. This can unfortunately be said for all anti-incontinence operations, however.

Paraurethral Injections

Some patients with dysfunction of the internal urethral mechanisms are candidates for the direct injection of material into the paraurethral (immediately adjacent) tissue, to deliberately cause a partial obstruction. Various materials are used for this, including some materials foreign to the body, but some natural materials like collagen are also used. Although quite simple and relatively easy, these procedures may have to be repeated a number of times, especially with collagen injections. Total obstruction and difficulty with voiding are possible problems, although these are potential problems with *any* of the surgical methods. Unfortunately, this is an expensive method depending on insurance coverage and it is not easily available in Canada. It is usually performed in patients where previous surgeries have failed, and who have urethras that have little or no function beyond being a fixed and dilated tube. It is ideal for medically unhealthy patients who are considered anesthetic risks, since it is quick, can be done under local anesthetic with little discomfort, and presents no problems with recovery from surgery.

Future Developments

New ideas are developed all the time. An interesting one that I've discovered utilizes various modalities of energy (freezing, radiofrequency waves, etc.) applied to paravaginal (pubocervical) fascia to cause it to contract and to pull up the urethra and bladder neck. Various techniques accomplish this laparoscopically, through open incisions or even vaginally. Simplistically, I think of these as methods to weld the paravaginal fascia back to the lateral attachment it has been torn from. Only time will tell whether these procedures will be successful.

Complications of Surgery

Surgery for incontinence may cause new problems. The elevation of the bladder neck, the inflammation of the healing process and the presence of foreign suture or sling material may all contribute to the development of an unstable bladder, even to the point of causing urgency incontinence. Although usually temporary, it may sometimes be a long-term problem that necessitates medical management. Fortunately, there is excellent medication available to us, which treats this effectively in most patients. Injuries to the bladder, the two ureters, or the urethra are possible, although not common, and can occur even when the most experienced hands have done the surgery. Some of these injuries might necessitate further surgery to correct. Urinary obstruction postoperatively is extremely common, but is usually only temporary. Prolonged urinary drainage by catheter or intermittent catheterization is sometimes necessary. Another possible complication that has to be mentioned is the increased incidence of enterocele formation after some bladder suspension operations. This usually occurs some time later, but there is no doubt about the increased long-term risk for this problem. Enteroceles will be discussed in chapter 11. Surely I do not have to say much about the possibility of bleeding, infection, and anesthetic complications. These are possible complications of all major surgeries. Insertion of foreign sling material will increase the risk.

Rest assured that all is not doom and gloom. Most patients will have an excellent surgical result, with either complete cure or a significant improvement in their urinary incontinence. Many patients start living again to their full potential after successful anti-incontinence surgery, and these women are usually some of the most grateful patients.

Notes

1. Arthur Bloch, "First Law of Scientific Progress," in *The Complete Murphy's Law* (New York: Price Stern Sloan, 1991), p. 130.
2. Bloch, "Whole Picture Principle," in ibid., p. 126.

TEN
Anal Incontinence

"My life has changed dramatically," says Stephanie, a marathon runner and fitness professional. "Exactly two years ago, during a vaginal delivery of twin boys, I experienced a fourth-degree tear. A year after that I had an external repair of my rectal sphincter. The doctors told me that less than 50 percent of my internal sphincter layers are left. Sometimes I have rectal bleeding, and frequently while jogging I will lose stools unknowingly. Is there any hope that one day I will be able to run farther than five miles without incontinence? My life is so altered with having to plan my bowel movements daily and never knowing when the next accident will be. I can only imagine what may happen when my twin boys want to go out or go on vacation, as their mommy is so embarrassing."

Although illustrating the indignities of anal incontinence with examples is clearly unnecessary, Stephanie's story is real and it should be told. It is obvious that any significant incontinence of stool or gas will have a severely negative influence on the quality of life.

It is estimated that up to 10 percent of women suffering from urinary incontinence also have anal incontinence. The National Institutes of Health (NIH) states that even though incontinence of gas (flatus incontinence) may be as bothersome as infrequent incontinence of stool (fecal incontinence), it is often discounted, a fact which may account for a significant underestimation of the prevalence of anal incontinence. For example, the overall prevalence of fecal incontinence has been reported to approach 20 percent, while the prevalence of fecal or flatus incontinence in a studied population of women following vaginal delivery was between 12 and 39 percent.

Anal incontinence could be considered the greatest closet issue of them all. Since it is considered to be a more socially unacceptable condition and generates more embarrassment than almost any other medical condition, it is seldom admitted to, even during visits to physicians.

I often find that patients tend to admit to anal incontinence only toward the end of the consultation period, and only after I have asked the question a number of times, and have created a conducive atmosphere for its discussion. Occasionally though, patients are referred with this specific problem, and will immediately describe their problem in such graphic terms, that even I would blush. It becomes abundantly clear what impact anal incontinence has on normal interpersonal relationships and day-to-day peace of mind.

Anatomical Implications

To understand some of the causes of anal incontinence—those that arise from vaginal childbirth—we need to look at the anatomy again. Certainly very few people actually stop to think about the processes involved in our ability to control our excretory organ systems. From an anatomical standpoint, bowel control is extremely fascinating, particularly since the continence mechanisms have to distinguish between different states of matter. The contents of the sigmoid colon (the lower part of the large bowel) include not only solid fecal matter, but also water and various amounts of gas. Normally we are able to distinguish the difference. The ability to pass gas without simultaneously passing liquid stool illustrates the amazingly intricate control we have.

As with urinary control, there are involuntary and voluntary mechanisms, which include the sphincter muscles and parts of the levator ani muscles. Similar to the bladder neck, the sphincters consist of an external (outside) and an internal (inside) sphincter, with only the external sphincter under full voluntary control. Again, reflexes play a major role in the constriction of these sphincters and muscles during sudden episodes of increased intra-abdominal pressure. Again, remember the pelvic floor trampoline model illustrated earlier. The main part of the pubococcygeus muscle illustrated is also called the puborectalis muscle. The name implies that the muscle has something to do with the pubis as well as the rectum, and that is exactly the case. This part of the levator ani muscle originates from the pubic bone, loops around the rectum, and implants in the pubis again. The pubic bone is the bone palpable underneath the mons pubis (area underneath the sexual hair), above and behind the clitoris. When it contracts, it pulls the rectum forwards and kinks it, which is one of the most important parts of fecal continence control. An intact and strong levator ani muscle with normal innervation is essential for this mechanism to work effectively. The puborectalis muscle could, with some justification, be said to be an extension of the external rectal sphincter. One does not usually contract without the other, especially not during voluntary contractions, as they are innervated by the same nerves, and are contiguous (fibers of the one flow into the other).

Normal continence not only depends on intact sphincters and pelvic floor muscles, but also on intact sensory mechanisms. It is

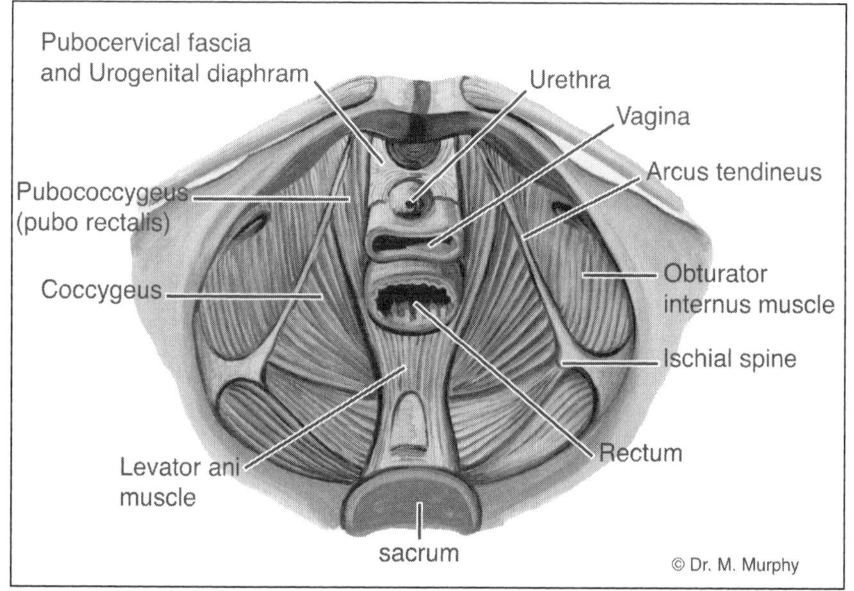

extremely important to be able to discriminate between solid stool, liquid stool, and gas. It should hardly be necessary to explain why this is important. All of us pass gas throughout the day, usually (if our continence mechanisms are intact) when we think nobody else will hear or smell. It is interesting to consider that the abhorrence toward the passage of bodily gases in public is a purely cultural development. Our ability to pass gas (only) safely, without a really bad accident (losing liquid or solid stool at an inopportune time), depends on the ability to perceive that it is only gas that is about to escape, and to prevent the escape from happening if not in a socially acceptable position, or if there is perceived uncertainty about the content. This amazing ability is the result of a process called "sampling." What in effect happens, is that the puborectalis muscle sling and internal rectal sphincter relax every now and then (up to seven times per hour), allowing the bowel content to descend into the lower rectum, close to the anus, where there are numerous nerve endings. These nerve endings are exquisitely sensitive and able to distinguish the bowel content. If they perceive liquid or solid stool, and the situation is not appropriate, the internal sphincter, and the puborectalis muscles contract again, sending the rectal content back up, till the next sampling.

These nerve endings can sometimes get damaged during a hemorrhoidectomy that is not carefully performed. This could lead to a "sensory loss" anal incontinence on the basis of a lack of discrimination of bowel content during sampling. Similar problems could occur with diseases, for instance Crohn's disease, although these inflammatory bowel diseases have many other reasons for bowel dysfunction, diarrhea, and incontinence.

Bowel distention by gas, fluid, or solids, will cause the sampling reflex to be even more active. During the relaxation of the internal rectal sphincter and the puborectalis, continence is assured solely by a strong contraction of the external rectal sphincter. It stands to reason that a weak or damaged external rectal sphincter could lead to incontinence problems.

Anal Sphincter Injuries

From the above, it is clear that the anal sphincters are essential to anal continence control. Injury to this sphincter is regrettably one of the most common injuries sustained during vaginal childbirth. In fact, detected via internal ultrasound, injuries to the anal sphincters have been demonstrated in up to *44 percent* of women after delivering their first baby. The incidence of fecal urgency or anal incontinence has been found to be as high as 20 percent; and although most patients recover, many find that problems persist, with up to 2 percent of women remaining completely incontinent for flatus (gas) or feces. The strength of voluntary anal sphincter contractions was found to be persistently low after vaginal delivery, both immediately postpartum and two months later. Those unfortunate women who develop rupture of their anal sphincters during birth have an increased chance for ongoing symptoms of anal dysfunction and incontinence (up to 50 percent of those with significant rupture, even with adequate repair). Studies differ widely in their findings, but overwhelming evidence points to a significant risk of prolonged problems.

Episiotomy

Until recently, episiotomies were done in an attempt to prevent vaginal tears and, especially, anal sphincter tears. Episiotomies have since fallen into disfavor as it was discovered that they do not successfully prevent bad tears. Although this has been adequately confirmed in large studies, most obstetricians will agree that episiotomy still has a place in modern obstetrics. Episiotomy can certainly shorten the second stage of labor in some patients, and may also prevent some of the nerve-injuring distension of the perineum right at the end of labor. However, it is equally true that episiotomy may lead to the transection of some nerve fibers.

No doubt the incredible stretching that the vagina and perineum undergo impresses anyone who has observed childbirth. It is *this* stretching that is considered so damaging to the pudendal nerve and which can also lead to tears of the pelvic fascia. During birth, the vagina and perineum not only stretch by dilating, but as a result of the downward forces, the perineum also bulges downward. Earlier on I discussed the rectovaginal septum, which anchors the perineum and prevents it from collapsing downward under the influence of gravity and intra-abdominal pressure. The forceful stretching during childbirth sometimes tears this important part of the pelvic fascia, causing a loss of perineal support. This, in turn, leads to excessive perineal bulging and secondary pudendal nerve injury.

The external anal sphincter is innervated by the pudendal nerves, which as we already know, are at risk during delivery. Partial denervation of the pelvic floor, usually involving the pudendal nerve, has been shown in up to *80 percent* of women after delivering their first baby.

Tearing

Perineal tears during vaginal birth are so common as to be more the rule than the exception. This is especially true in primigravidas (first-time moms) and it is usually impossible to predict in whom perineal tears will occur. Fortunately the tears often involve only the mucosal lining (moist skin layer) of the vagina and is then classified as a grade-one tear. If the tear involves the underlying muscle of the vagina, or even the pelvic floor muscle, it is classified as grade two, whereas a tear of the external anal sphincter is a grade-three tear. If the tear is even more extensive and has torn right through the vagina into the bowel, including a total disruption of the external anal sphincter, it is a grade-four tear. As already mentioned, a very high percentage of women sustain injuries to their anal sphincters that can be demonstrated by ultrasound or other sophisticated techniques. However, most of these are not clinically appreciated.

It is the responsibility of the caregiver to suture these tears in an anatomically correct way that reconstitutes the different layers. As a result of the significant swelling, bruising, and distortion of the tissue planes as well as the concurrent bleeding immediately after childbirth, it is sometimes quite difficult to do just that. Improperly or hastily repaired tears or episiotomies can lead to long-term disability, which may include incontinence or pain during intercourse. As with most surgeries, the first repair is the most important. All subsequent attempts will have to contend with scarred, denervated, and devascularized tissue (tissue that has lost its normal nerve and blood supply). The latest information on the suturing of episiotomies indicates that there might be some advantage to leaving the outside skin layer open, rather than suturing it. Although this flies in the face of conventional wisdom, it seems this might lead to fewer wound breakdowns, possibly related to a decreased incidence of hematoma formation (blood clot entrapment). Suturing of episiotomies has traditionally been seen as a training area for young physicians. With our current knowledge of the importance of correct repair of episiotomies and vaginal and perineal lacerations, this attitude is definitely not appropriate anymore. Suturing the vaginal epithelium after a few sutures have been thrown into the muscle is not sufficient. A serious attempt needs to be made to find the underlying fascia defects that have been created, and correct them. In order to do this appropriately and to understand what you're actually doing and why, significant knowledge of the anatomy, as well as the physiology and pathophysiology of pelvic floor disorders is required.

One simple example of how the lack of a sufficient basis of knowledge leads to inadequate management can be found in the routine suturing of external sphincter lacerations. Many practitioners will make the correct diagnosis, and proceed to suture the external sphincter appropriately, usually end to end, but will do so for a total width of probably 5 mm, or maybe 1 cm. This is in spite of the fact that the external rectal sphincter is approximately 2.5 cm wide! I can speak from personal experience that this knowledge had been quite a revelation when I first became aware of it, as nobody had ever taught me this. I cringe when I think back on the hundreds of "5 mm–1 cm" sphincters I've sutured.

Other Factors Related to Damage

A few other factors have been shown to increase the risk of injury to the pelvic floor and the anal sphincter muscles. These include multiparity (more than one baby), big babies, instrumental delivery (by forceps or obstetrical vacuum), a prolonged second stage of labor, an abnormal position of the baby during delivery, and a history of a previous injury incurred during childbirth. It has been found that forceps delivery is significantly associated with an increased risk of pelvic floor injury. Vacuum extraction seems to be significantly safer in this regard. Unfortunately, instrumental vaginal deliveries cannot be totally eliminated. By allowing a much longer second stage of labor, the incidence of instrumental deliveries can and has been decreased; but it is now suspected that a prolonged second stage is another significant risk factor. This is often disregarded by the natural childbirth movement, but it is likely that many of its supporters are simply unaware of the facts. Most of the consequences of a damaged pelvic floor usually show up years after childbirth, and it is difficult to get excited or overly concerned about a remote possibility in the face of one of the most emotional, exciting, and significant moments of a person's life.

Surgery for Anal Incontinence

Surgery for anal incontinence generally involves repair of the perineum and the external anal sphincter. The surgery is often done immediately postpartum if a sphincter or perineal laceration is identified. Incontinence however usually implies previous injury and the surgery is thus done electively (at a predetermined date) at a later stage.

Most authorities agree that a previous injury associated with anal incontinence symptoms puts a women at great risk for a repeat injury to the anal continence mechanism. Consequently, there is significant risk of symptomatic anal incontinence. The first surgery for any incontinence or prolapse situation is always the most important, since subsequent surgeries have a much lower success rate. Therefore, elective cesarean is recommended for women during a subsequent pregnancy after any previous successful anti-incontinence surgery.

ELEVEN
Genital Prolapse

Leslie is a thirty-five-year-old mother of a one-year-old son, her only child. Soon she'll undergo surgery for prolapse, which has caused her pelvic organs to protrude outside her body. "It's hard to lift my son because the body parts come out. It's like half of a ping pong ball slipping out," she explains. Leslie deals with the problem by pushing the organs back in place. "Before the birth of my child, I never heard the words cystocele, rectocele, enterocele, or pelvic floor. I did learn those words at my six-week postpartum checkup. I've spent the last eight months getting second and third opinions from surgeons and researching all the aspects of this all-too-silent issue," she says.

The word "prolapse" comes from Latin, and means "to fall." Prolapse literally involves a situation where organs fall or descend past their normal positions. Genital prolapse, or otherwise called pelvic organ prolapse (POP), can involve any of the main pelvic organs including the bladder, uterus and cervix, and the bowel. Women suffering from genital prolapse often have associated urinary or anal incontinence, although it is urinary incontinence that is most prevalent. Difficulties or inability to void or have bowel movements are also common. Other symptoms are dependent on the specific abnormality, but usually include a feeling of pelvic fullness or discomfort, lower back discomfort, or the appearance of a bulge in or even out of the vagina. Also prevalent are symptoms of vaginal laxity, lack of sensation during sexual intercourse, and general genital discomfort. If the prolapse is severe enough, the friction of the mucosa (vaginal tissue) to clothes can lead to itchiness, bleeding, and infection. I have also had the occasional patient that complained of severe pelvic pain, which is usually not caused by pelvic prolapse.

Uterine Prolapse

With significant uterine prolapse, the uterus sometimes protrudes completely out of the body. When standing, this causes significant discomfort, and women usually have to push the organ back in before they can sit down. Even in lesser degrees of uterine prolapse the feeling of vaginal fullness can be extreme. The lower parts of the uterus and cervix often become swollen and this, together with continual scratching on clothes, pads, and panty liners, can cause an ulcer to develop, which can bleed or cause a discharge. Although this severe degree of prolapse (called total procidentia) is by no means rare, the more usual degree of uterine prolapse is far more moderate. It would involve the uterus and cervix moving up and down in the vagina (almost like a piston in a sleeve). Uterine prolapse could also often cause sexual dysfunction in the form of dyspareunia (painful intercourse). Downward movement of the uterus pulls the upper vagina with it, and creates traction on the bladder base. This may cause the impression of a cystocele (bulging of the bladder), and can also cause bladder irritability that could lead to symptoms of overactive bladder. Additionally, as a result of the displacement of the bladder, the bladder neck, and the urethra, stress urinary incontinence is often associated. One has to remember that uterine prolapse most often occurs concurrently with global pelvic floor damage, which is often related to dysfunction of other parts of the pelvic floor. As such, uterine prolapse is often combined with various forms of urinary incontinence, anal incontinence, as well as other prolapse problems of the rest of the vagina.

Uterine prolapse is the result of damage to the support structures at multiple levels. By now you are familiar with the levator ani muscles and the pelvic fascia as support structures. Uterine support, in addition, involves certain specific ligaments and is dependent on a normal uterine position in the pelvis.

The uterus is usually tilted and bent forward in such a way that when one is standing, its long axis is lying almost horizontally. In this position, the shelf of the levator ani muscles and the pelvic fascia support the bulk of its mass. In some women the uterus is bent backward and, although this is less common, almost the same applies. The uterosacral and cardinal ligaments are specific ligaments attached to the lower part of the uterus and to the pelvic sidewalls. These ligaments are usually very strong and provide significant support to the uterus.

Damage to the pelvic floor leads to an increased aperture of the opening that the vagina and cervix penetrate (the urogenital hiatus), which as we know is the result of weak, wasted, or torn levator ani muscles and pelvic fascia. In the setting of stretched or weak uterosacral and cardinal ligaments, it is not surprising that the uterus would simply slide down through this opening. It is really a simple matter of gravity—if the anchors of the uterus fail and the underlying support is weak, the uterus *will* descend.

As mentioned before, all the pelvic support structures are less rigid and more pliable in pregnancy, which explains to some degree the occurrence of uterine prolapse in some women even during their first pregnancy. Of course, the added weight of the fetus and increased uterine weight are significant cofactors in the development of this problem, but fortunately, as the uterus enlarges it reaches a point where it is too large to move through the pelvis. This solves the problem for the moment, although such women are at higher risk for a recurrence during future pregnancies, and I would consider them to be at higher risk for future pelvic organ prolapse.

Diagnosing uterine prolapse is usually a relatively simple matter. Many women have told me that they are feeling something hard in the vagina. I clearly remember one young woman who told me that she was feeling a "bone" coming through her vagina! The point is that the cervix can often feel quite firm, and most women can clearly feel their cervix when putting a finger into the vagina. In more severe cases the cervix can be seen protruding downward, or even through the vaginal opening when using a hand mirror. When it protrudes right outside the body, the diagnosis is obvious. In these

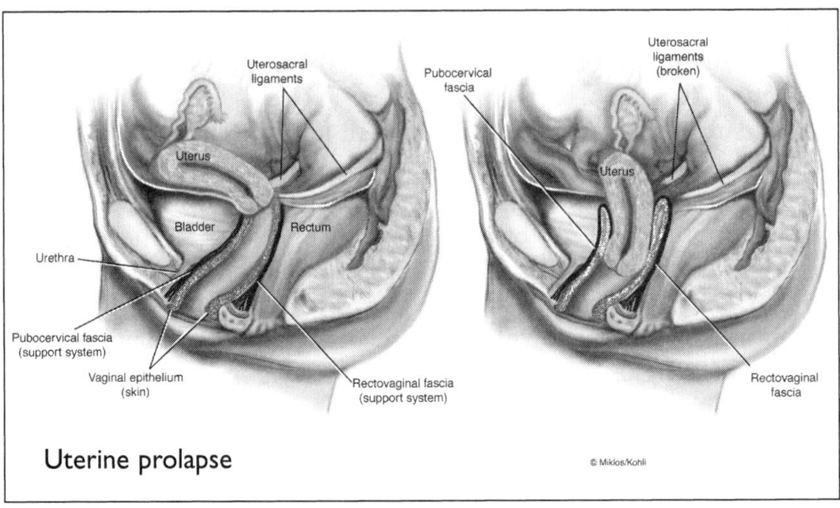

Uterine prolapse

cases the prolapse always involves descent of the bladder and bowel. When experiencing symptoms that might be related to prolapse, it is very important that the physician examine the patient not only supine (lying on her back), but also standing erect. It seems that some physicians have not taken Newton to heart, and are ignoring gravity, to their patients' detriment.

There is one condition that can simulate uterine prolapse, but has a totally different origin. These are cases of cervical elongation, a situation where the cervix is elongated to the point where it appears low down in the vagina. As a result of its position in the vagina, symptoms mimic those of uterine prolapse. Cervical elongation is often an incidental finding during examination for other conditions. Its presence can cause substantial difficulties during a vaginal hysterectomy, and may require the gynecologist to convert to an abdominal procedure.

Vaginal Vault Prolapse

Vaginal vault prolapse is the prolapse of the vagina after previous hysterectomy. This condition is often misdiagnosed as a cystocele or rectocele. Complicating matters, however, is the fact that these conditions often occur together. Treatment for vaginal vault prolapse is basically the same as for uterine prolapse.

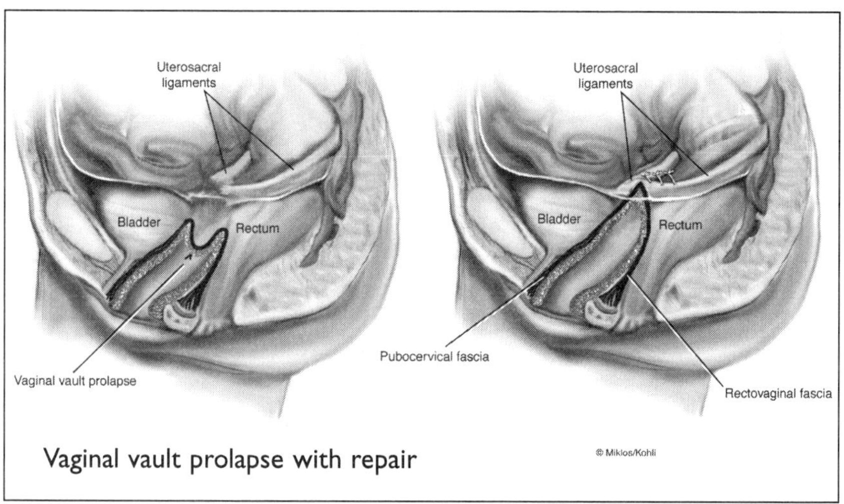

Vaginal vault prolapse with repair

Cystocele

A cystocele is an abnormal bulging of the bladder into the vaginal roof (anterior vaginal wall). This is experienced as a bulge in the vagina from the top, which sometimes comes right down to the vaginal entrance and even through the entrance. The anatomical defects are by now familiar. These, not surprisingly, involve torn or fractured pelvic fascial layers, ruptured fascia ligaments, or levator ani muscles weakened by one of the factors discussed earlier.

Cystoceles are commonly accompanied by urinary incontinence as a result of bladder neck support deficiency. For a cystocele to develop, the backstop support must be deficient. If you think back to the garden hose example in the development of stress urinary incontinence, the reason for the association of urinary incontinence and cystoceles become more understandable. Urinary incontinence does not always occur in the setting of a cystocele however, so it is sometimes difficult to understand why some patients are totally dry in the presence of an obvious cystocele. The answer of course is that the backstop support is not the only factor important to continence. There also are the internal and external urethral sphincters, which have already been discussed.

Some very large cystoceles mask the incontinence problem by kinking the urethra, by virtue of their extreme prolapse. This could in the long run lead to renal (kidney) problems resulting from recur-

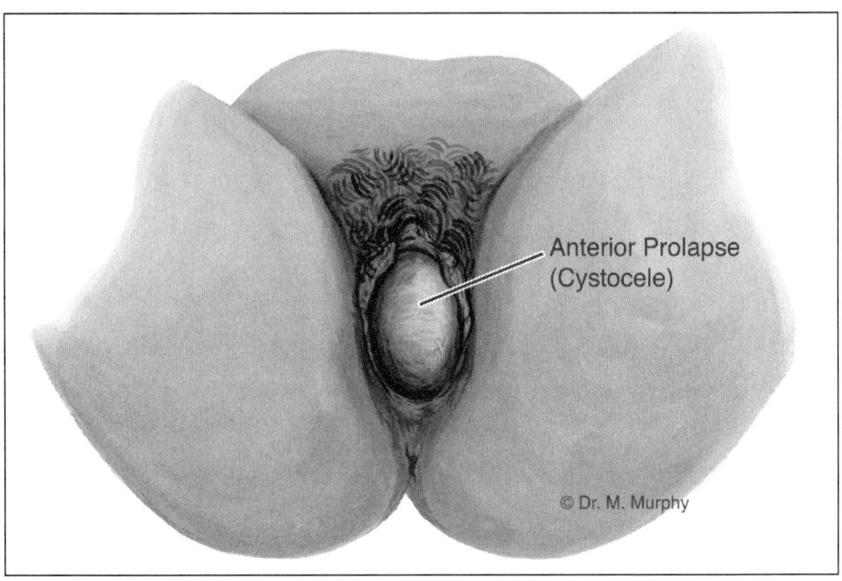

rent infections, or increased backpressure on the kidneys. Curing cystoceles via surgery sometimes has the unfortunate side effect of unmasking the stress incontinence. So while the patient is cured of her cystocele, she is not much better off, and often not happy at all. Such patients invariably consider the surgery as having been a failure. I have found this to be a problem when counseling patients preoperatively. It is an extremely important concept for patients to understand, even if only for purely selfish reasons on the physician's part. Today's expectation is that outcomes should all be perfect. We find the same attitude in obstetrics, where if the outcome is not perfect (for instance, having a perfect baby) there is a tendency to want to blame somebody. This "somebody" is usually the health care professional and this results in an absolute explosion in health care-related litigation. So it is essential to discuss the possibility of latent (hidden) incontinence preoperatively. If this is not done, and stress incontinence develops after a technically perfect antiprolapse surgery, the surgeon is sure to be blamed for having caused the incontinence. But note that simply discussing the possibility is not good enough. The physician should at least try to find out how likely this is to happen, and modify the surgical approach if necessary to include an anti-incontinence procedure. This can be accomplished to some degree by reducing (pushing in) the prolapse—the cystocele or uterine prolapse—and then letting the patient cough or perform other activities that usually bring on stress urinary incontinence, with a full bladder. It is best if this is performed erect, rather than lying down. There is no point doing this with an empty bladder either, so I usually perform this test immediately after my office cystoscopy, when there is a known volume in the bladder. The prolapse can be reduced either manually, or with a pessary.

Although doing this will pick up many cases of latent incontinence, it will not diagnose it in everybody, which is the point that needs to be stressed. The bottom line is that occasional patients, where latent incontinence was not expected, might require a future procedure for stress incontinence should this develop after corrective surgery for prolapse. However, it is the surgeon's responsibility to think of this possibility when planning the surgery.

Consider that most so-called cystoceles are nothing of the sort. A real cystocele is a herniation of the bladder through a tear in the midline fascia, and can be diagnosed cystoscopically as a downward bulging of the bladder wall. It is now recognized that many, if not most, anterior vaginal wall prolapses, which had in the past been diagnosed simply as cystoceles, are really cases of paravaginal defects. What happens here is that the pubocervical fascia has torn away from arcus tendineus fascia pelvis (also called the white line of the pelvis) on either or both sides, which then leads to a downward

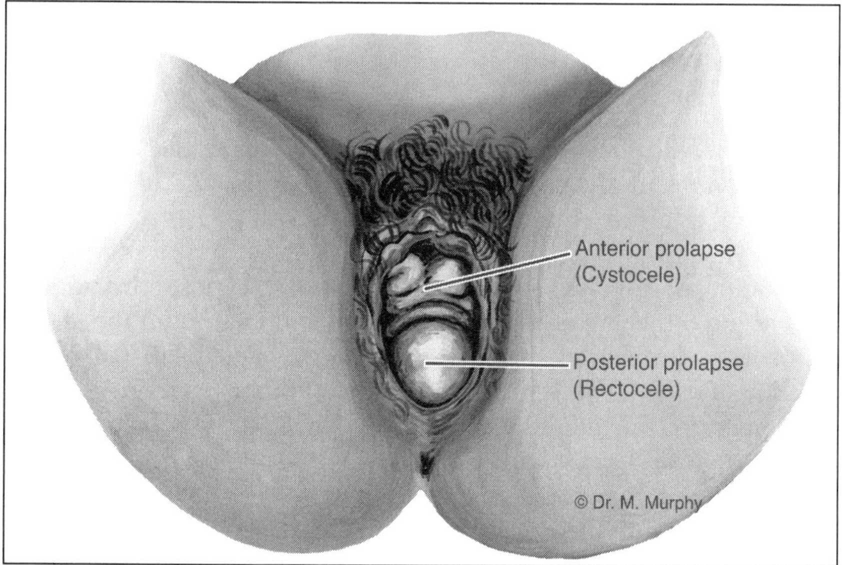

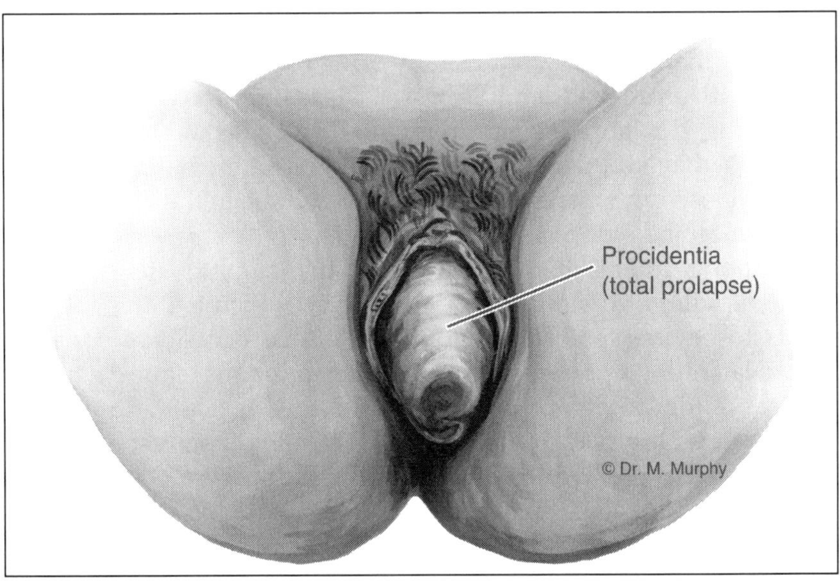

movement of the entire anterior vaginal wall. The bladder, resting on and supported by the anterior wall, simply moves downward, without any true herniation. The correct diagnosis in these cases is paravaginal defect(s), not cystocele. The implications of misdiagnosis will lead to inappropriate and eventually unsuccessful surgery.

Rectocele

Rupture of the rectovaginal septum could lead to bulging of the rectal wall into the vagina. This is called a "rectocele," and often occurs as a result of weakened levator ani muscles and an increased urogenital aperture (the openings in the pelvic floor perforated by the urethra, vagina, and rectum). The bulge might be low down in the vagina or involve the whole length of the posterior vagina, depending on where and how extensive the damage and the tear(s) in the fascia layers are. This rectal bulge can almost be visualized as a ballooning of the bowel into the vagina with the resultant effect of fecal material collecting in this pouch. Patients often complain of constipation, and a need to reduce the vaginal bulge by putting their fingers in their vagina to assist defecation. Others have noticed that they need to splint their perineum with their fingers, in order to pre-

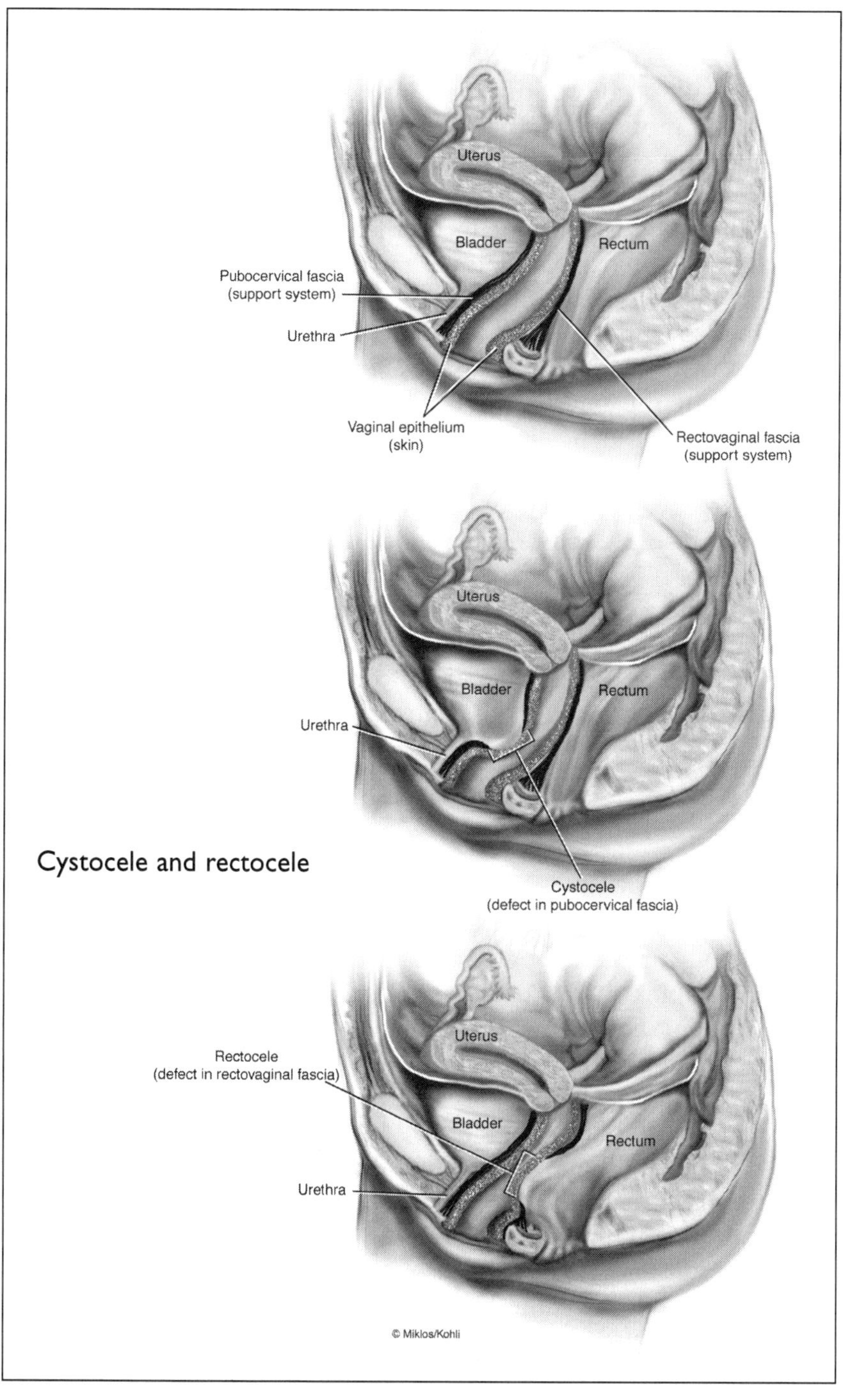
Uterus
Bladder
Rectum
Pubocervical fascia
(support system)
Urethra
Vaginal epithelium
(skin)
Rectovaginal fascia
(support system)
Uterus
Bladder
Rectum
Urethra
Cystocele and rectocele
Cystocele
(defect in pubocervical fascia)
Rectocele
(defect in rectovaginal fascia)
Uterus
Bladder
Rectum
Urethra
© Miklos/Kohli

vent excessive downward bulging of the perineal area, and to assist in bowel evacuation. This downward bulging of the perineum is another result of the rupture of the rectovaginal septum. Excessive downward movement then secondarily leads to progressive pudendal nerve stretch injury, giving rise to a vicious circle.

In lesser degrees the resultant fecal collection might cause a feeling of pelvic fullness or incomplete bowel evacuation. Just as cystoceles are often associated with urinary incontinence, rectoceles are often associated with various bowel function abnormalities, including constipation and fecal or gas incontinence. Rectoceles often occur in the setting of associated perineal body injury, often with injury to the external anal sphincter. It is obvious that in those cases, anal incontinence is likely.

Just as in cystocele, the fascia (rectovaginal septum) tears can occur in various areas. If there is a localized tear, a localized bulging will be the result. Repair of these localized tears is called "site-specific repair."

Unfortunately, the association between the anatomy and the function of the rectum is less established than that of the bladder. It is difficult to predict the functional outcome of surgery for posterior vaginal prolapse and posterior compartment pelvic floor dysfunction.

ENTEROCELE

The intra-abdominal space between the lower part of the uterus, vagina, and the rectum is called the "pouch of Douglas." Usually this space is functionally obliterated by the position of the vagina, since the vagina in the usual situation is in an almost horizontal position (lying flat against the pelvic floor). Usually there is no real "space," just a potential one.

If for some reason this space opens up, it will immediately fill up with bowel loops, since it is situated low in the pelvis and the bowel loops will naturally move there under the influence of gravity. The most common reason for this to happen is a rotation of the vagina from its horizontal position to a more vertical position. This is usually the result of a weak pelvic floor. It also frequently occurs after hysterectomy, if the vaginal vault was not suspended from the uterosacral ligaments in the normal position.

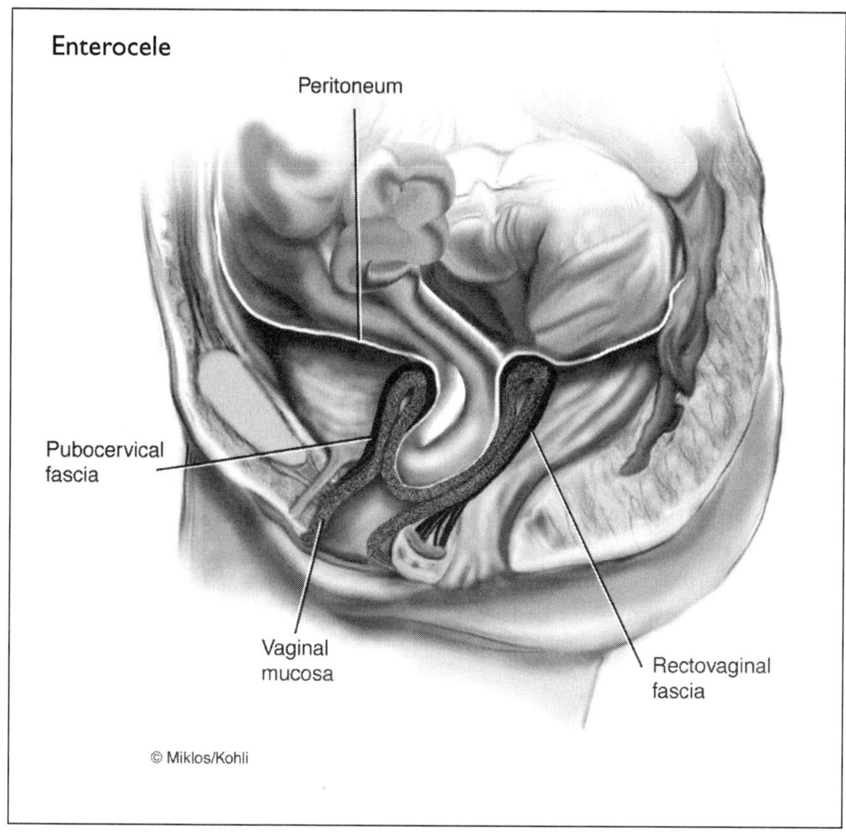

An intact rectovaginal septum is also important to ensure the integrity of the separation between the intra-abdominal cavity and the vagina. A torn or weakened fascia, especially the rectovaginal septum, could lead to the formation of a hernia through the weakened upper part of the posterior vagina (back wall of the vagina).

Most people are aware of groin hernias, which form when the intra-abdominal contents bulge through a weakened lower abdominal wall, causing a noticeable, uncomfortable, and often painful swelling. These groin hernias may contain only fluid or fat, but sometimes they contain bowel loops. In the same way, a weakened posterior vaginal wall could lead to hernia formation. If the vagina is in the normal horizontal position, this will not happen, since no forces are exerted on the posterior wall. If its axis changes, as described above, so that the forces of gravity are directed toward the posterior vagina, a weakened fascia (in this case rectovaginal septum) leaves only a weak separation between the intra-abdominal contents and the vaginal cavity. The only remaining layers that then separate the inside of the vagina from the bowel loops are some fatty tissue, the vaginal mucosa, strands of muscle, and the intra-abdominal lining (peritoneum). In time this will stretch out and form a pouch that bulges into the top of the vagina. This might likewise contain only fluid or fat, but often it contains loops of small bowel. If severe, this hernia (called an enterocele) could fill the whole vagina and even bulge through the vulvar opening to the outside of the body.

Since their origins are entirely different, it is important for the gynecologist to carefully distinguish between an enterocele and a rectocele during physical examination. Enteroceles are commonly missed during examination for genital prolapse and this could (not surprisingly) lead to early recurrence of prolapse problems after surgery if not found and corrected at the time of surgery. I know from personal experience in my more timid days, that gynecological surgeons are often faced with a situation where it is difficult to decide whether the bulge encountered after dissection of the rectovaginal space—to correct a rectocele—is an enterocele or the rectum itself. I can think back on many occasions where I chickened out, persuading myself that the bulge was the rectum itself, and then proceeded to correct the supposed rectocele. The reason for this is that if one cuts into the rectum itself, it could have nasty consequences. In cases where this was indeed an enterocele, the patient is sure to have less than optimal outcomes, often to return with continued or renewed bulging, and all the symptoms associated. If my own experience is to be taken as representative, I believe there are thousands of women undergoing rectocele repairs where enteroceles are not diagnosed. This might be part of the reason why surgery for rectocele is often not associated with symptomatic improvement.

Through trial and error I have learned to become more aggressive in opening these pouches, to look for enteroceles. There is, however, the occasional moment of trepidation prior to cutting, and I have probably lost a few years off my lifespan as a result. I can still remember the saying of one of my wise and experienced older teachers in South Africa. Prior to making these incisions, he would pause for a few moments, and then in an almost prayerlike voice, make the following statement: "Boldness, be my friend."

One possible way to overcome this problem is to perform

barium meals and defecography. These are tests where barium is placed into the rectum and sigmoid through an enema, and a barium meal is taken as for other upper bowel radiological investigations. X-ray studies are then performed during straining, as well as active defecation. The barium meal is required since enteroceles often involve the small bowel, whereas rectoceles involve either the rectum or sigmoid colon. It is clear that these tests are quite unpleasant since I have yet to meet somebody who enjoys defecating in public. They are thus not commonly performed. They are also expensive and will contribute to ever increasing wait times for radiological procedures and surgical treatment itself.

Rectal Prolapse

Similar processes to those described above can lead to rectal prolapse. This occurs when the rectal tube slides through the anal canal

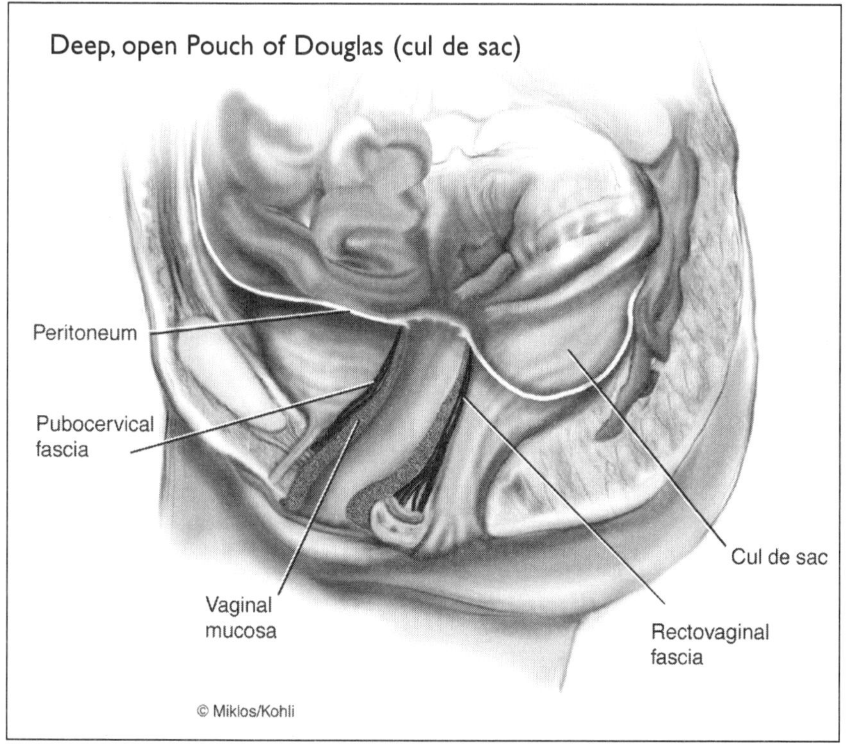

and protrudes outside the body. The normal rectal position is also dependent on intact pelvic support mechanisms. Fortunately, it is the least common pelvic prolapse problem, and if present it is usually minimal. Distinction must be made between rectal mucosal prolapse only, and full thickness bowel prolapse. Full thickness prolapse is the result of intussusception. This occurs when the bowel folds into itself. Mild degrees of intussusception might also be a cause for bowel-related symptoms from rectoceles, only to persist after surgical correction of the rectocele. Intussusception can only be diagnosed by barium studies or direct endoscopy, for instance sigmoidoscopy (that is where a doctor looks into the rectum and sigmoid colon) and as a result I suspect they are often missed, especially if mild.

Significant rectal prolapse is almost uniformly associated with some degree of anal incontinence, or other symptomatic rectal or anal dysfunction.

TWELVE
Treatment Options for Genital Prolapse

I am a thirty-eight-year-old woman dealing with a partial prolapse that seems to be getting worse. I think it was caused by the forceps, the very long labor, and a nine-pound baby. I've been to the gynecologist and she said I seem on the borderline for surgery. The procedure would entail cutting a piece out of the vagina and shoring it up, providing a resting place for the bladder. As I live in Britain, there are waiting lists. I am to hang on as long as I can cope. Can physical therapy cure a partial prolapse, one in which there is only a tiny protrusion out of the vagina? Since diagnosis, it is slipping further out. Is it better to leave it alone? Should I be concerned about a long wait for surgery? I can imagine that the remaining muscles might be getting a bit fed up.

From a posting on www.pelvicfloor.com

As with urinary incontinence, treatment options for genital prolapse include surgery or more conservative methods. But unfortunately, because pelvic organ prolapse is usually the result of anatomical changes related to damage and weakness of pelvic floor support tissue, conservative methods are used mostly to postpone inevitable surgery or act as a substitution for surgery that is too risky or not even possible. It is important to note that pelvic organ prolapse does not always require interventional treatment options, specifically surgery, just because it is present. Some patients seek only an explanation for their symptoms, and hopefully this book will contribute in that regard. Others want the problem fixed and, for most of them, that will require surgery.

Pelvic Floor Exercises and Genital Prolapse

Although some might disagree, I am of the opinion that pelvic floor exercises have little direct value in the treatment of moderate to severe genital prolapse. Since pelvic fascia tears and ligament weakness are almost always present, strengthening the pelvic muscles, even if possible, is seldom effective in treating the existing prolapse. This is different from urinary incontinence, where I believe strengthening the levator ani and sphincter muscles may have definite value and should often be the first thing tried. Yet pelvic floor exercises are always a good idea as even if unhelpful in treating established prolapse, they curb further muscle deterioration and prevent other pelvic floor disorders.

Thinking back on the anatomy and physiology of the pelvic floor, the reader will remember that if the pelvic floor muscles become weak, the full brunt of the strain lies on the connective tissue layers (fascia). So, in time it is inevitable that the prolapse will worsen. Strengthening the muscles via pelvic floor exercise will protect the fascia to some extent by taking up some of the strain. It will *not* cure the tear in the fascia.

Pessary Effectiveness

Pessaries are devices placed in the vagina (see also page 82) and although effective in some women, are not very popular. Reasons for this may include the gynecologist's unfamiliarity with pessaries, the reluctance of patients to accept them, and the existence of more effective surgical treatments. In properly selected patients, pessaries can have a very significant and beneficial role to play. I am referring here to the frail, older, sedentary patient who may be unwilling or unable to safely undergo major surgery.

Pessaries can also be used in pregnancy, especially during the early months of pregnancy if significant prolapse occurs before the natural enlargement of the uterus resolves the problem (often only temporary). Another place for pessaries is in the preoperative period, to help heal ulcers on the tip of the prolapsed cervix and to decrease the swelling of the prolapsed organs. Some women are so uncomfortable during this waiting period that a pessary could bring welcome temporary relief.

The choice of the correct type and size from the several types of pessaries available is more art than science, and experience is achieved only by trial and error. It often comes down to fitting various types and/or sizes to see which works best. Some of the factors that need to be taken into account are whether patients are sexually active, or are dexterous enough, and physically able to reach into the vagina. These factors will all play a role in the decision regarding which type of pessary to use, or whether attempted pessary use is even appropriate. Some pessaries can stay in for months at a time without removal or cleaning, whereas others (for instance the cube pessary) need to be removed daily for cleaning.

For safe usage of a pessary, vaginal atrophy needs to be prevented or treated if present. For patients not on systemic hormone replacement therapy, some form of occasional vaginal estrogen might be required. One of the simplest ways to accomplish this is to use an Estring. This is a soft silicone ring that contains estrogen, and that releases the estrogen slowly over the course of three months. The hormonal concentrations are so low that it has minimal effects on the rest of the body, but it is sufficient to prevent atrophy of the vaginal and urogenital tissues. These rings can be left in the vagina for the three months without the need for removal for cleaning, and sexual activity is not precluded with them in place. However, they can be removed, cleaned, and later reinserted. It is really easy to do. Estring is ideal to use with one of the pessaries that can stay in for a long time, such as a ring pessary, but can also be used with any other pessary as a less messy alternative to estrogen vaginal cream.

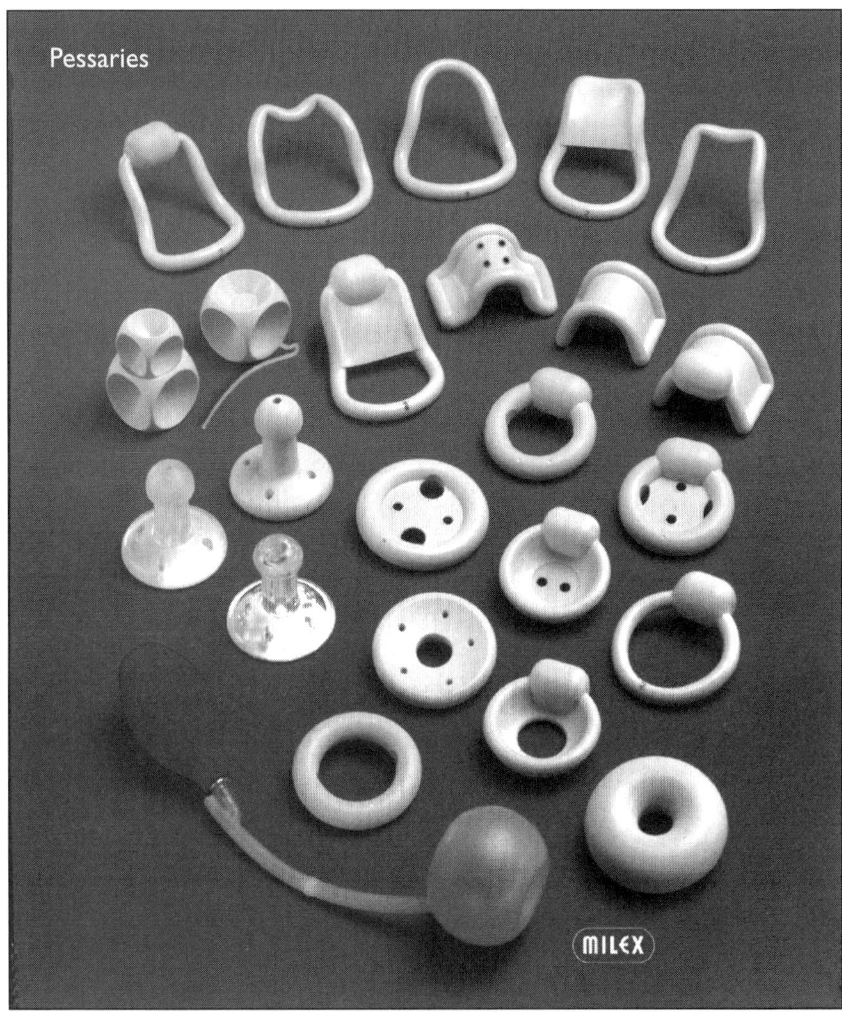

Ask Questions Before Surgery

The mainstay of treatment for genital prolapse is surgery. The finer aspects of specific surgical procedures are beyond the scope of this book, but I will briefly explain some of the general concepts. Although some of these concepts may seem difficult to understand, the purpose is to arm women with enough information so that they can cover any pertinent questions and concerns prior to any surgical procedure.

HYSTERECTOMY AND UTERINE PROLAPSE

Many gynecologists still believe, especially with regard to uterine prolapse, that simply removing the offending uterus will cure the problem. This may certainly be true in the immediate short term, but there is an excellent chance that these patients will be back for further management of their ongoing, but now differently manifested prolapse problems. Many of these physicians assume that the patient is suffering from a new problem, since from their perspective, the patient had already been cured of her uterine prolapse. In truth, it is the *cause* of the prolapse that has to be identified and repaired at the time of the initial surgery. In other words, it is obvious that the pelvic fascia must be repaired, where defective, and the vagina must be suspended from secure structures for future support.

PREVENTING PROLAPSE AFTER HYSTERECTOMY

After hysterectomy, the vaginal vault (that is, the innermost part of the vagina, formed by suturing the cut surfaces of the vagina after removal of the uterus and cervix) needs to be attached to something; otherwise there is a risk of future prolapse, especially when there is preexisting lack of support. Simply leaving it hanging there without adequate support is asking for trouble.

In many cases of hysterectomies for prolapse, the structures utilized for this suspension function are the so-called uterosacral ligaments (see illustrations on page 137). These ligaments are very important in the support of the uterus in all women, and weakness could contribute to pelvic organ prolapse problems. If these ligaments were strong, uterine prolapse may not have happened in the first place. Many gynecologists, however, continue to use only the ends of these structures as the only means to support the vaginal vault. It comes as no surprise, then, that the recurrence rate of vaginal prolapse is high after hysterectomies performed for uterine prolapse.

The Mayo McCall Suspension Procedure

The uterosacral ligaments can be utilized very effectively for support during pelvic floor reconstructive surgery if done correctly. This is the basis of the Mayo McCall suspension.

The Mayo McCall culdeplasty procedure (its full name) is my preferred suspension operation. Popularized by the Mayo Clinic, it is the suspension procedure most endorsed by its pelvic floor surgeons. With experience, it is relatively easy to perform. In contrast, I find the sacrospinous ligament suspension (also called the Richter suspension procedure, discussed next) is quite difficult. The Mayo McCall culdeplasty creates excellent, strong, and, in my view, anatomically superior results. The procedure can be done after hysterectomy to suspend the vault and prevent future prolapse, or to treat existing prolapse. It can also cure and prevent enterocele formation. It can even be used with the uterus in place, where preservation of the uterus is required or preferred. Simplistically, the procedure consists of suturing the uterosacral ligaments together in the midline, and suturing the vaginal vault to these uterosacral ligaments. Importantly, the sutures are placed high up in the deep pelvis, through the substantial body of the uterosacral ligaments and through the obturator muscle fascia and not through the ends of the attenuated ligaments where cut from the cervix. A number of sutures (up to four or five) are sewn to create a strong suspension. At the same time, the apex of the vaginal vault is tapered slightly to prevent the formation of a broad area on which intra-abdominal forces are directed.

Discuss the Risks of the Mayo McCall with Your Surgeon

The most significant risk with the Mayo McCall culdeplasty procedure is trauma to the ureters. The ureters run just above the area where the sutures need to be placed, and there is a risk of them being encircled or punctured. As a result, intraoperative diagnostic cystoscopy with confirmation of ureteric patency is essential after this procedure so that offending sutures can be removed if necessary. This can easily be accomplished by injecting a blue dye intra-

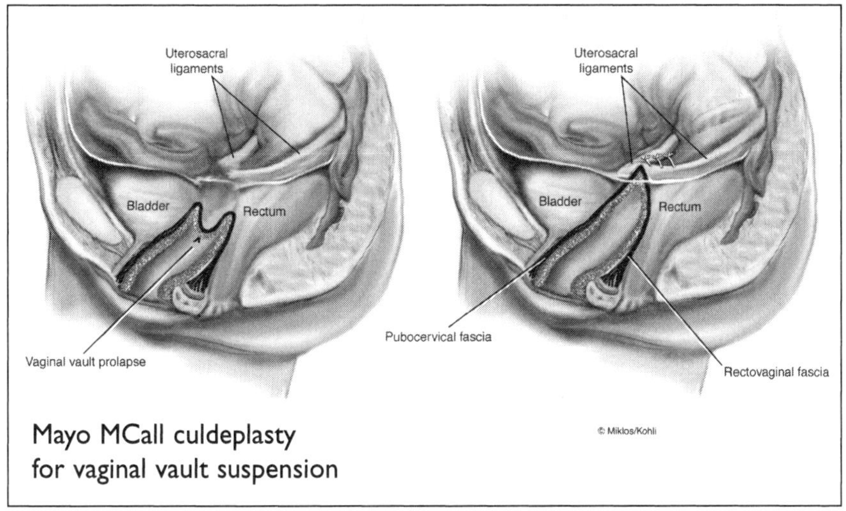

Mayo MCall culdeplasty for vaginal vault suspension

venously, which is excreted by the kidneys into the urine, and then observing the dye coming through the ureteric orifices in the bladder. Ever wondered why your urine was blue after pelvic surgery?

Diagnostic cystoscopy has been a problem for some gynecologists in hospitals where it is preferred that urologists perform them. It is another example of interspecialty rivalry for personal agendas, and where patient-focused perspective is lost. Diagnostic cystoscopy after difficult pelvic surgery, for exclusion of bladder trauma and confirmation of ureteric patency, is becoming the standard of care, and in my view, is not optional. Neither is it appropriate to call a urologist for each and every case.

Sacrospinous Ligament (or Richter) Suspension Procedure

You may have correctly deduced that the most commonly performed surgical procedures for uterine prolapse include hysterectomy. In the absence of contraindications, this can be done as a completely vaginal procedure with no abdominal incisions. To prevent future vaginal vault prolapse, a variety of other suspension procedures could be performed. One mentioned earlier is the so-called sacrospinous ligament (or Richter) suspension procedure. The sacrospinous ligament is obviously used here as the strong point.

Although this is a very effective method, it does have disadvantages. It necessitates a somewhat more substantial dissection in the pelvis than vaginal hysterectomy alone, with resultant risks of damage to blood vessels or pelvic nerves, or injury to the rectum. Such injuries could be very difficult to manage as a result of the deep locations of the affected structures in the pelvis. Sacrospinous ligament fixation also causes the vagina to be in a slightly off-center position, which might lead to future problems, including increased cystocele formation. It requires special instruments that are not always readily available, creating added expense. It does restore the horizontal position of the vagina (albeit not exactly anatomically correctly), which decreases the risk of future enterocele. Sacrospinous ligament fixation has been found to have no significant influence on sexual function, which was an earlier concern with this procedure. It also has the potential to cure prolapse with preservation of the uterus, although that is not commonly performed. This procedure is in some cases combined with a repair of the rectovaginal septum to cure or prevent a rectocele.

Overall, I believe the Mayo McCall procedure is the better procedure. It is quick, requires no special instruments, and could be done almost as part of a vaginal hysterectomy. It adds only a few minutes, creates excellent and strong anatomical support, and has few risks provided ureteric patency is confirmed. As with most situations in surgery, there will be many different opinions. It often boils down to which procedure the surgeon feels more confident doing, and has more experience with.

Uterine Removal After Prolapse

This is a complicated issue. As I indicated, I believe that in many cases of uterine prolapse, the removal of the organ is considered the entire treatment of the problem. Now it is clear that this is a fallacy. Removal of the uterus does nothing to correct the underlying pathology that led to the prolapse.

However, in most cases of *significant uterine prolapse*, removal of the uterus is indeed preferable during corrective surgery. Thus it is part of the cure, but not the whole cure. The uterus often acts as a weight, pulling down on the vaginal vault, exacerbating the preexisting weakness, and increases the risk of recurrence of prolapse. However, uterine preservation is possible in some cases, and of course, in younger women for whom fertility is an issue, it becomes imperative to preserve the uterus. Procedures like the Mayo McCall culdeplasty, or sacrospinal ligament fixation could be utilized to correct uterine prolapse while leaving the uterus in place. If pregnancy follows successful pelvic floor reconstructive surgery, elective cesarean birth should be seriously considered.

Surgery for Vaginal Vault Prolapse

The surgical treatment for vaginal vault prolapse is similar to that of uterine prolapse. Both the Mayo McCall culdeplasty, as well as sacrospinal ligament fixation procedures could be employed. A totally abdominal approach is often used for correction of vaginal vault prolapse. The abdominal approach could be through an open laparotomy, or by laparoscopy. The benefits of the laparoscopic approach include the lesser invasiveness and quicker recovery. In this respect it is similar to the pros and cons of laparoscopic approaches to urinary incontinence treatment. The abdominal (open or laparoscopic) procedures often utilized include sacrocolpopexy, an abdominal procedure analogous to the Mayo McCall vaginal procedure. The vaginal vault or cervix is sutured to the bodies of the uterosacral ligaments and obturator fascia. Sacrocolpopexy involves suspending the vaginal vault from the longitudinal ligament in front of the sacrum, by using an intervening mesh. Basically, one end of a piece of mesh is sutured to the abdominal side of the vaginal vault (or uterosacral ligaments if the uterus is present and is to be preserved), and the other end is sutured to a strong ligament that runs down the front of the spinal column. Since this ligament as well as the mesh is very strong, a very strong suspension can be obtained. In fact, this procedure provides the most secure suspension of the vaginal vault. There are problems with the procedure, however. Mainly, these include the approach (abdominal rather than vaginal), and the choice of the mesh material and potential complications of its usage. There are numerous kinds of mesh materials that have been discussed in the urinary incontinence section. The same problems previously discussed in chapter 9 apply here.

SURGICAL REPAIR FOR CYSTOCELE AND RECTOCELE

The surgical steps for the repair of cystoceles and rectoceles are similar. The vaginal mucosa (vaginal skin) is opened, and the fascia is sutured, after which the mucosa is trimmed and then resutured.

For decades, there has been a debate regarding whether the rectovaginal fascia between the vagina and the rectum (in cases of rectocele), as well as the pubocervical fascia between the bladder and the vagina wall (in cases of cystocele), can actually be seen during surgery in a live patient, in contrast to surgical dissection in cadavers, and whether breaks in this fashion can be identified.

Some researchers insist that no distinction can be made between the vaginal wall muscle fibers, and this so-called fascia, whereas others vociferously defend this belief. The idea of site-specific repairs is that individual fascia tears can be identified, isolated, and repaired. I have to admit that I'm a fence sitter on this one. Although I do believe that I have often found what appear to be tears in the support structures, I do have difficulty identifying individual fascia tears. I believe some of the so-called tear identification is a combination of a bit of wishful thinking and the need, induced by the competitive academic environment in some institutions to agree that, indeed, the problem was found, identified, and fixed. I am not at all implying that our concept of the pelvic fascia, and the damage to it, is incorrect, or that surgical repairs should not attempt to fix or reinforce this fascia. I just don't believe that one can always clearly see the tears.

More recently, abdominal methods of repairing these two defects have become popular. These include the paravaginal repair as described in chapter 9.

Enteroceles are usually repaired at the time of rectocele repair. The hernia sack is opened, tied off, and the opening through which the hernia occurred is repaired.

A relatively recent development is the incorporation of mesh patches in cystocele and rectocele repair. The significant failure rate of standard repairs has increased the search for the ideal mesh material. Unfortunately, the ideal mesh has not yet been found, or developed. All meshes have potential problems or complications, but in cases of previous failed surgery, it is becoming more common to utilize mesh. This is because there is often no visible support tissue to be found with which to accomplish a repair that has any likelihood of long-term success.

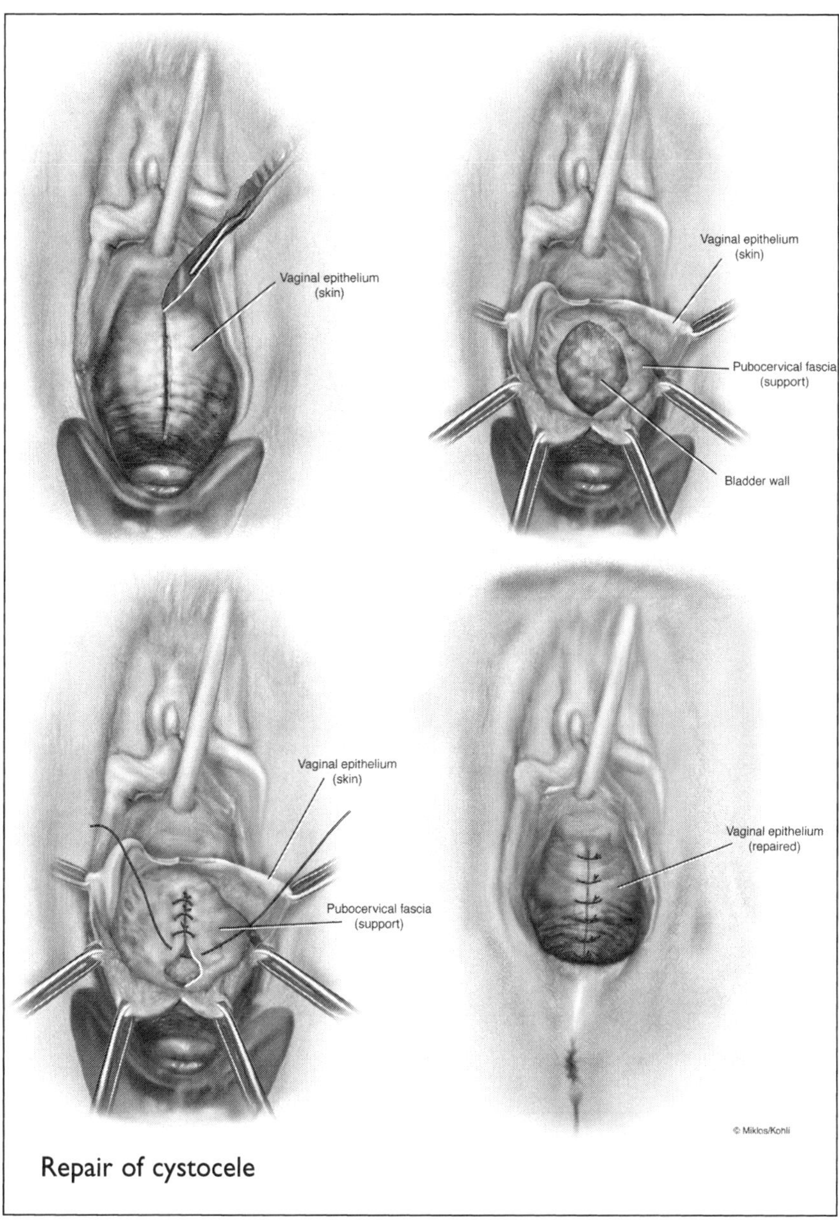

Repair of cystocele

One further surgical procedure that is occasionally performed is the so-called LeFort colpocleisis. This is a procedure where the vagina is basically sown shut. Rest assured that this procedure is recommended only for the extremely frail, medically unhealthy, or

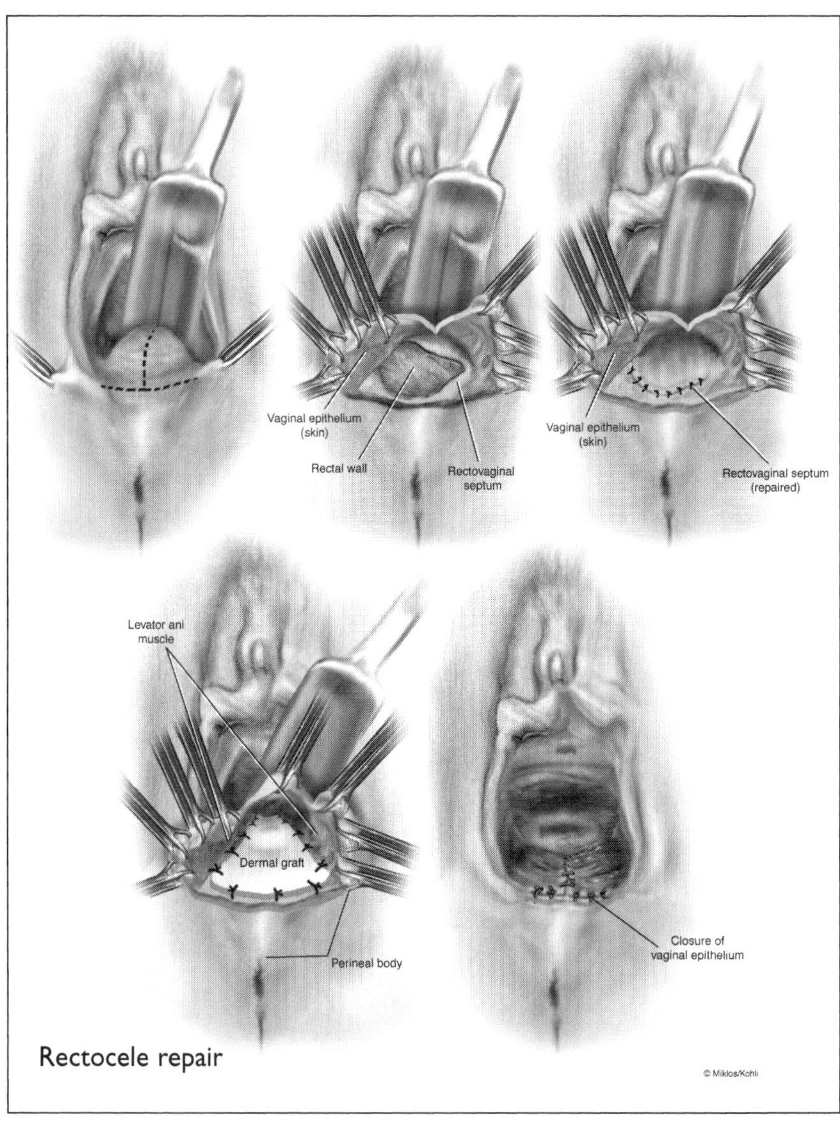

Rectocele repair

older patient where coital function is not an issue. Strips of vaginal skin are removed from the upper and lower walls, after which the surfaces are sown together. This has the effect of shutting the vagina, preventing the organs from falling through the genital opening, which now doesn't exist, but leaves small drainage canals on each side for the secretions. The reason this procedure is preferred in such cases is that it is quick and can be performed under local anesthetics

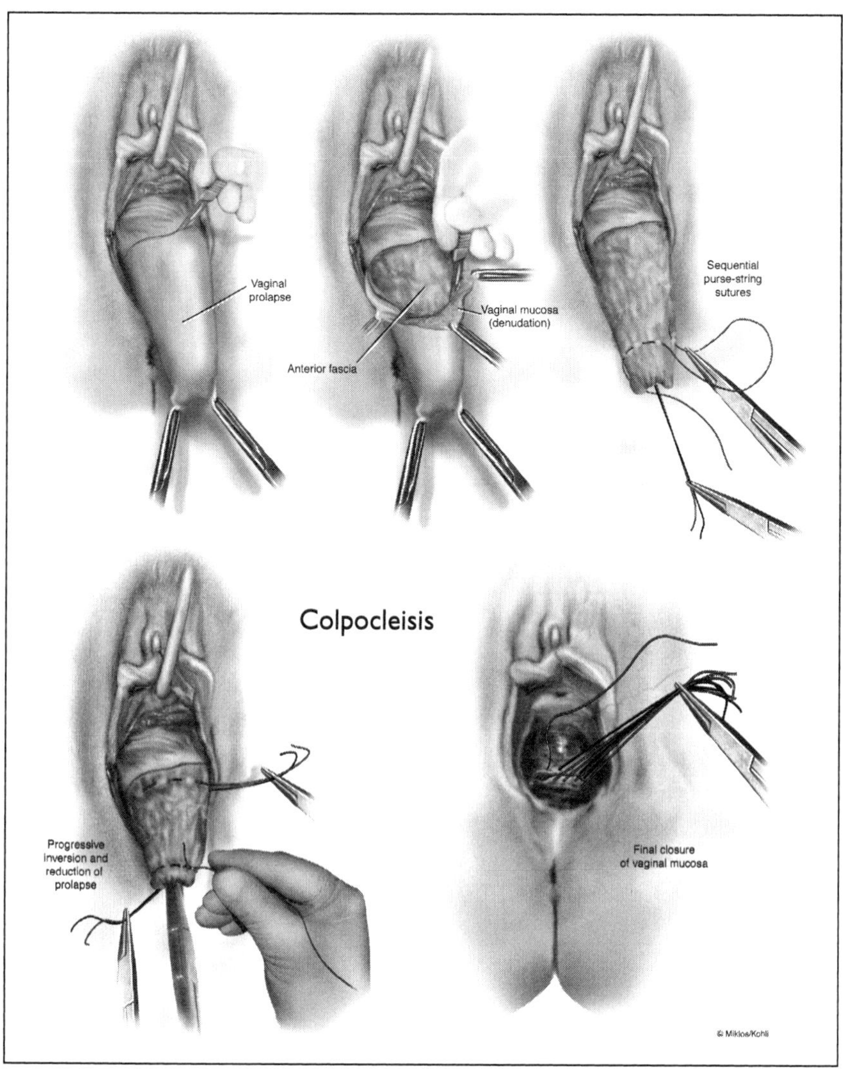

with some sedation. The likelihood of significant complications is also reduced.

EXAMPLES OF SURGICAL COMBINATIONS

Here are just a few commonly occurring defects and combinations of defects, and some suggested combinations of treatment procedures that are often performed together. It is by no means an exhaustive list.

- **Uterine prolapse, cystocele, rectocele, stress urinary incontinence:** Vaginal hysterectomy, TVT, anterior and posterior repair and McCall culdeplasty, or sacrospinous ligament fixation.
- **Uterine prolapse, paravaginal defects, rectocele, stress urinary incontinence:** Vaginal hysterectomy or laparoscopically assisted vaginal hysterectomy with McCall culdeplasty, or sacrospinous ligament fixation, laparoscopic paravaginal repair and laparoscopic Burch, then vaginal rectocele repair. These same procedures can be done through open laparotomy (open abdominal hysterectomy with modified McCall culdeplasty, open paravaginal repair with open Burch, then vaginal rectocele repair). This will take a lot less time than the laparoscopic procedures.
- **Paravaginal defects:** Laparoscopic or open paravaginal repairs (with or without adding Burch sutures to treat existent or latent stress urinary incontinence).
- **Uterine prolapse with need or wish to preserve uterus:** Laparoscopic or open (by laparotomy) modified McCall suspension, or laparoscopic or open sacrocolpopexy with mesh (suspension of cervix to presacral ligament using mesh interposition). A vaginal sacrospinous ligament fixation or McCall can also be done. I have had good results with vaginal McCall uterine suspensions.
- **Vaginal vault prolapse:** Sacrocolpopexy (open or laparoscopic), McCall culdeplasty or sacrospinous ligament fixation. There are almost certainly other defects as well that will have to receive attention at the same time. These could include anterior repair (cystocele), posterior repair (rectocele), and treatment of latent or overt stress urinary incontinence by for instance Burch colposuspension, TVT, or some other sling procedure.

From the above combinations, it is obvious that there are a great variety of procedures that the surgeon will have to consider based on an assessment of the underlying pathology, specific problems, and a history of previous surgery. After previous failed surgery, some procedures might be technically very difficult to repeat, and others are more likely to fail and would thus be inappropriate. The use of mesh is also more likely to be required to affect a strong repair.

During any posterior repair, the perineal body might need to be built up again (perineoplasty), and the external rectal sphincter might require attention. As mentioned, mesh support could be integrated into the repair process of almost any of the above-mentioned procedures. Various mesh products are available, none of them ideal, and individual gynecological surgeons and urogynecologists will make their decisions on what is available, cost factors, personal preferences, and company support.

One of the principles of pelvic surgery is that the whole pelvic support structure has to be seen as one entity. It's almost like a house of cards. Shoring up only one wall will not prevent the house from collapsing. The whole pelvis needs to be evaluated and considered for treatment. It is well known that correcting some defects could directly increase the risk of other defects developing, or increasing in severity. Some classical examples are the Burch colposuspension, which increases the risk of posterior defects like enterocele, and the sacrospinous ligament colpofixation, which increases anterior defects such as cystocele.

I'm not saying that *every* little bit of organ descent needs to be repaired! Pelvic surgery by its very nature could lead to possible further neurogenic damage and has the potential for further muscular dysfunction and weakening of the pelvic floor. The gynecologist/urogynecologist must have the ability to decide what is indeed a real problem in terms of the whole structure, and what is incidental and insignificant. Although this sounds like a relatively simple matter, it can become very complicated and difficult to make those decisions. It often becomes art, rather than science, and there is no substitute for real-world experience, in contrast to book knowledge and the hand holding nature of teaching hospitals.

THIRTEEN
Complications of Pelvic Floor Surgery

When talking about complications after pelvic floor surgery, it is extremely important to clarify just what we are talking about. There is a big difference between a less-than-ideal outcome, and an unintended complication such as bleeding or trauma to an adjacent organ. It must be said that patients' expectations play a large part in their perception of the outcome, and this is outside of the surgeon's control.

As far as outcome is concerned, the exact final result is always an open question, and cannot be predicted. One thing is certain: After having children, a woman's vagina and her pelvic floor support will never again be *just* as it was before. Not to say that a woman must ever merely *settle* for a lesser quality of life—no—but most of us, perhaps grudgingly, do acknowledge the realities of the aging process. No surgeon, whether the most well known or the most influential, can ultimately change that.

Surgeons will not know exactly how things will turn out, even though they wish for the best and may give the impression that there is an exact expectation. Since pelvic floor reconstructive surgery often involves the "whole house of cards," not all the parts may be perfect afterward. As emphasized, sometimes the act of fixing one problem unmasks another defect that was hidden and unknown. Also, for reasons we've discussed, one or more of the corrected problems may recur.

Surgeons Are Human

The more surgery a surgeon does, the more complications that surgeon will get. This is a fact of life, regardless of how good the surgeon is. *All* surgeons get complications. *All* surgeons are human. Equally important—*all* patients are human. We are *all* human, and as a result, things do (relatively often) go wrong. Yes, there is a vast difference between complications caused by negligence and those resulting from the normal course of practice and contingency. Unfortunately, patients often find differentiation difficult in this regard. When things do go wrong, it is easy for an adversarial relationship to develop between the physician and the patient. Certainly, today's medical versus legal controversies have negatively affected patient/physician relationships. Needless to say, there are always bad apples in the world that need to be exposed and stopped. But arguably, patients will experience more harm than good in societies where the practice of medicine is beleaguered by overzealous legal systems and adversarial physician/patient relationships.

Common, but Often Temporary Complications

Urinary function might change after pelvic floor surgery, especially if an anti-incontinence procedure was done. First, there could be the inability to void altogether. This is usually managed with a catheter but more appropriately with intermittent catheterization. Although initially hesitant, this is something that most patients can easily learn. Dependent on the procedure, this is usually only necessary for a few days, with the occasional patient having to continue for more than a week. Even after this, there is the possibility of permanent changes to the urinary stream. Often it takes longer to start, and the stream is slower. Occasional patients find they can only urinate standing up, or leaning forward (usually temporary). There is the possibility of overactive bladder symptoms after surgery. This is usually temporary, and if of longer duration, can often be alleviated with anticholinergic medication.

Constipation is a common postoperative problem. Factors responsible include opiate medications for pain that are known to cause constipation, but also the immobility that is common after surgery. Major surgery sometimes leads to "ileus." This is a situation where the bowel is "paralyzed" temporarily, and distends significantly with retained fluid and gas. This is related to a functional obstruction versus a true obstruction, which is most often the result of adhesions.

Additionally, a patient might be disappointed that her vagina is somewhat different. It may not be as tight as she expected or hoped it would be after surgery, or she might complain that it is too tight. It might be shortened. There might be some extra mucosal ridges or tags, roughness, or even scar tissue that patients might find aesthetically displeasing, or sexually uncomfortable.

Bleeding

Bleeding is a complication. It can happen acutely, during surgery, or later on. Arteries or veins can tear, slip out of sutures, or be missed by sutures or clamps. Sometimes during vaginal surgery where traction has to be exerted to enable one to reach the vessels, they might slip, and retract to above the area where one might be able to see, or reach. Sometimes these same vessels go into spasm and do not bleed at the time, only to bleed later on, long after the patient is back in the ward. More acute intraoperative bleeding can also occur. This might necessitate immediate laparotomy (opening up) during a vaginal hysterectomy, or necessitate various procedures to control bleeding during open or laparoscopic surgery. Acute active bleeding during a laparoscopic procedure will also sometimes necessitate opening up (laparotomy) to be able to evaluate and deal with the problem. Slow bleeding could give rise to blood clots (hematomas) accumulating somewhere in the abdominal cavity, or in other cavities where work was done. These hematomas might require drainage or evacuation.

Active bleeding in a patient that is otherwise stable could potentially be managed with embolization of the offending vessel. This is a procedure where an interventional radiologist threads a catheter through a patient's femoral artery from the groin and then selectively finds the bleeding vessel by injecting contrast material and watching with fluoroscopy (X rays). Various plugging materials could then be placed into the bleeding artery, which obstructs the artery and stops the bleeding.

Acute, life-threatening bleeding during surgery often requires clamps or sutures to be placed in somewhat more haste than would otherwise be the case. This could potentially lead to the next step in the vicious circle, for instance injury to the ureter.

Ureteric Injury

Ureters are the muscular tubes carrying urine from the kidneys to the bladder and are *always* at risk during almost *all* pelvic surgical procedures.

A little inside-the-specialty saying: Pelvic surgeons, we say, are "married" to ureters. We think of them constantly. We fear them and we love them. When we don't see them we fear for them. When we see them we love them. It's like a marriage.

The ureters not only course through the entire pelvis, but they also cross immediately under the uterine arteries (main feeding arteries of the uterus), wrap very close to the cervix on their way to the bladder, and lie only about 1 cm above the uterosacral ligaments. They can be difficult to see, as they are only about 4 to 5 mm in diameter, covered by peritoneum, and are the same color as all the other structures. This is especially true if there is distortion of the normal anatomy as a result of a disease process (for instance endometriosis or infection). They can also be located in unusual positions, for instance when pushed away from their normal course by fibroids or ovarian cysts. So, there are numerous possible causes for injury to the ureters, or for clamping them, or for encircling them with sutures.

The most important thing regarding ureteric injury (other than preventing it) is to diagnose it as soon as possible. If this is not done, kidney damage could result. I have already discussed one way of confirming ureteric patency after difficult pelvic surgery (cystoscopy with indigo-carmine dye intravenously; see chapter 11 for treatments for genital prolapse). When doing abdominal surgery, whether laparoscopic or open, one can dissect the ureters free of the surrounding tissue, and follow their course through the pelvis under direct vision. Unfortunately, such dissection carries some risk of the injury that one is actually trying to prevent. Postoperatively, one could do an IVP (intravenous pyelogram), which is a test where radio-opaque dye is injected intravenously and excreted by the kidneys into the urine. X rays will then hopefully confirm ureteric patency.

INFECTION

Another common complication is infection. The vagina is not a sterile place. There are billions of bacteria in the vagina, just as for instance in the mouth. No amount of cleaning or antiseptic solution will change this fact. Any surgery done in or through the vagina thus has the potential complication of an infection. This is of course true for any surgery and according to legal practices in Canada at least, does not even have to be mentioned as a potential complication after surgery, since any reasonable person knows this.

However, after pelvic floor surgery it is important to note that the risk may be higher in light of a number of factors. First of all, patients might have difficulty urinating after the operation, which could lead to urinary tract infection. Second, there might be some pooling of blood in the pelvis after a hysterectomy especially, which could easily lead to a pelvic infection or abscess formation. Since the vagina is full of bacteria, as well as its proximity to the rectum and anus, infection after vaginal surgery itself is also more common. Having said all of this, however, it is remarkable how infrequently really serious infections occur.

INJURIES TO THE BOWEL OR BLADDER

Just as in the possibility of an injury to blood vessels or ureters, the same possibility exists for injuries to the bowel and bladder. The nature of pelvic floor reconstructive surgery is that one works in close proximity to, or immediately on, these structures. The separation between the surgical plane and the walls of these organs are often very difficult to see, and exceptionally easy to breach. Often the organs are stuck together with adhesions that need to be cut surgically in order to perform the required procedure. The normal anatomy is usually distorted, which is the reason for the surgery in the first place. The sequelae (what follows) from injuries to these organs depend on many factors. It could mean simple resuturing and leaving a catheter in for a few days, but it could also lead to the need for further surgical procedures immediately, or in the future. Occasionally, injury to the large bowel might require a temporary colostomy. The help of other surgical specialties such as colorectal, urological, or vascular is sometimes required.

Anesthetic Complications

As with any surgery, there are numerous potential complications related to anesthesia. Most are discussed in the section on possible complications after cesarean birth (see chapter 18).

Any major surgery, especially where general anesthetic is used, could also lead to lung complications such as pneumonia. It's important to breathe deeply in the postoperative period, to make sure the lungs fill totally with air. Incomplete lung expansion (atelectasis), as a result of shallow breathing is the main cause of most lung problems after surgery. Sometimes physiotherapy is required to help prevent lung complications.

Thromboembolic Complications

Mainly, thromboembolic complications encompass deep vein thrombosis and pulmonary embolism. These complications are discussed in chapter 18 and will not be handled here.

FOURTEEN
Pelvic Pain

"I have been to so many doctors since the pain started some three years ago," says a middle-aged woman in a letter to the International Pelvic Pain Society (IPPS). "A laproscopcy yielded nothing but a picture-perfect uterus. I had an appendectomy in 2001 as an effort to rid myself of a worsening nightmare of pain each month. I didn't know pain could be as bad as this. Every doctor in my area had given up on me," she remarks. Her happy ending, she says, is when she read about "conscious pain mapping" on the IPPS Web site. After consulting with a doctor familiar with the procedure, it was discovered that a hidden hernia was the apparent cause of pain. She still has some pain but to a much lesser degree, and she is being treated with medication. This patient is one of many who experience pelvic pain, and this is one of many ways to approach the condition.

The IPPS suggests preparing a pain diary prior to your first visit with your physician. Note the following information:

- Location of the pain (entry to the vagina, deep inside).
- Characteristics of the pain (dull, aching, sharp, etc.).
- When it happens (during sex, while sitting or standing, during the menstrual cycle).

- Triggering events for the pain, if any.
- What you do to cope with the pain (avoid sex, take pain medications, rest, exercise, etc.).
- Why you think you are experiencing pelvic pain.

According to a 1994 survey of five thousand women, eighteen to fifty years of age, 14.7 percent reported having suffered from chronic pelvic pain. Of those women, 15 percent had lost time from work because of pain and 45 percent said it had affected their productivity. In another study of about six hundred sexually active, menstruating women, 39 percent reported current pelvic pain.

Pelvic pain is incredibly common, could be debilitating, and is extremely difficult to diagnose and treat. It is always a great relief for the patient, and for the gynecologist, when an actual cause for the pain can be definitively identified, and when a specific treatment exists for the condition. But sadly, it is all too common that a cause cannot be clearly identified, or that a cause is found for which there is no proven and universally effective treatment. The wide range of possible culprits often makes it difficult to come to conclusions at the first or even second visit as to the cause of the pain, which sometimes creates an impression that either the doctor doesn't know what she/he is doing, or is not taking the complaints seriously. Trust me: This is not the case. As gynecologists, we see so many women with pelvic pain that we fully realize the complicated nature of the condition and the extent of disruption this nebulous entity creates in personal lives as well as in society. Unfortunately, the impact of the disorder doesn't make it easier to understand.

Many physicians feel a definite sense of dread when a patient mentions the "pelvic pain" phrase. It immediately conjures up images of time-consuming investigations, repeated office visits, a myriad of possible treatment combinations, and continually frustrated, unsatisfied patients.

Although I don't for a minute want to minimize this (I get the same feeling of resignation when I hear "the phrase"), I believe there are ways to make the whole endeavor less painful (pun intended). It requires a significant patient education effort, one that addresses the fact that as far as pelvic pain is concerned, things are often not what they seem. Patients *must* remain *open minded to all possibilities*.

Many gynecologists have given up on pelvic pain because the

underlying psychosomatic and psychosocial conditions that are very often the cause of the condition are difficult to find, and even more difficult to explain or to understand as potentially causal. The immediate negative reaction that many patients have when psychosomatic or psychosocial causes are brought up, or even hinted at, has the unfortunate effect of encouraging many physicians to steer clear of the subject altogether. The condition of pelvic pain is just loaded with minefields, especially for male physicians. The reason I say this is that pelvic pain, as is the case with many chronic pain conditions, often occurs in patients with significant underlying psychopathology. This is not always the case, or even the case in the majority. However, it is frequent enough to require consideration in *all* sufferers where another diagnosis has not yet been made.

For example, those with endometriosis or ovarian cysts have a recognizable cause for pain. When present, physicians can do what we are trained for—to investigate, diagnose, and treat. There is a problem, a definition, and an endpoint. We are comfortable.

With chronic pain without a recognizable finding, all bets are off. Many physicians immediately become insecure. There is no clearly defined problem. Everything is open ended. Single practitioners are at a definite disadvantage in terms of optimal care, since such patients are best managed by a multidisciplinary team that may include physicians, psychologists, physiotherapists, social workers, and others. Since the health care system in most countries is fragmented, this is seldom achieved.

Some physicians may deal with their insecurity, frustration, or lack of knowledge or resources by appearing less than empathetic. Patients may be told it's all in their head and feel that their problem is being dismissed as trivial. Other physicians may look for the quickest way to get rid of the patient by making the problem (or at least the complaints) go away temporarily. This often involves immediate referral out, or requesting investigation after investigation. After all, quickly scribbling on a lab requisition form takes a lot less time than really listening to the patient and doing a detailed physical investigation.

I once had a colleague who stated: "Our job as physicians is to amuse our patients until nature cures them." Although there is definitely a lot of truth to that statement, it shouldn't include losing empathy. Being up front about the fact that they don't want to deal with such problems is a legitimate choice that physicians can make, however. In such cases it would be better if the patient understands that from the beginning, so that appropriate referral can be accomplished to another specialist or to a clinic with such an interest or practice. If this is done as a policy (not ad hoc), it cannot be considered dumping, and patients should not perceive negative insinuations. I will mention that in Calgary, we are lucky to have such a multidisciplinary clinic. After the appropriate investigations have ruled out obvious physical diseases, patients can be referred there for multidisciplinary care from a team that can support each other and provide services and time that are impossible in the typical practice setting. This kind of clinic is often very expensive to establish and run. There are limited opportunities for private funding, and it works best in a socialized or at least government-supported setting, especially since many patients may be younger women with inadequate private health plans. At this point in time, our clinic's future hangs in the balance as a result of threatened funding cuts, proving again that pelvic health is not on the radar screen as far as priorities go. Despite the fact that the clinic is literally restoring a normal life to many women who are disabled by chronic pain, the bureaucrats can, and might, destroy it all by a flick of a pen.

Fortunately, there are many physicians with special training or an interest in chronic pain syndromes. Such physicians realize that defined physical diseases are but one side of chronic pelvic pain. Affecting each of us are the psychological, emotional, and social aspects that also need to be addressed, if only to get background information to formulate possibilities and hypotheses regarding all possible causes. As testing proceeds, these more subtle conditions are not forgotten.

Pelvic pain can be the result of numerous conditions, many of which fall outside the scope of this book. As such, I will just briefly discuss some specific conditions that may be more relevant, and will mention only a few additional possible causes.

Possible Causes of Pelvic Pain

This is not an exhaustive list and not in any order of importance or prevalence:

- Abdominal muscle strain/inflammation
- Adhesions from previous surgery
- Bladder disorders, such as interstitial cystitis or infection
- Endometriosis
- Fallopian tube disorders, such as infection or hydrosalpinx
- Hip or pelvic joint problems, for instance arthritis
- Incisional hernia
- Inguinal hernia
- Irritable bowel disease (IBS) and other bowel motility disorders
- Ligament strain/inflammation
- Ovarian disorders, for instance ovarian cysts or adhesions affecting the ovaries
- Pelvic floor muscle spasms (often in cases of vaginismus and vulvodynia)
- Pelvic inflammatory disease (PID) and sexually transmitted disease (STD)
- Pelvic organ prolapse
- Pregnancy or pregnancy complications
- Psychosomatic or psychiatric disorders
- Rectal/colon disease, for instance diverticulosis and inflammatory bowel disease (Crohn's/Ulcerative colitis)
- Referred pain from causes in other body parts
- Torsion (rotation) of the ovary, cyst, or fallopian tube (collectively known as the "adnexum")
- Uterine disorders, for instance adenomyosis or fibroids
- Various cancers
- Vulvodynia

Pain from Prolapse

Pelvic organ dysfunction and prolapse yield varying levels of symptoms, from no symptoms at all to severe symptoms that may become disabling. These could include urinary or fecal incontinence, urinary or bowel urgency and frequency, constipation, pelvic or back discomfort and pain, and paradoxically sometimes difficulty or even the inability to pass urine or bowel movements. An enlarged vaginal aperture in the setting of weak pelvic floor muscles can also lead to sexual dysfunction and dissatisfaction. And, as if this were not enough, pelvic organ prolapse can also cause pain. I've had the occasional patient who suffers with severe pelvic pain where prolapse is the only obvious finding. Not believing that it could be the prolapse causing the pain, I have investigated some of these patients with almost every method known to man, only to find nothing else at all. In some of these cases, the pain went away after the prolapse was repaired. I can immediately hear the skeptics saying, "placebo effect!" I'm still personally unconvinced that pelvic prolapse is a common cause of severe pelvic pain, but I'm slowly and grudgingly accepting that it can be. This is in line with some proponents of the so-called integral theory who suggest that many cases of pelvic pain could be related to damage to pelvic support structures, especially in the upper levels of the vagina. These researchers propose that repairing areas of vaginal relaxation could significantly improve, or even cure, many previously dismissed patients with pelvic pain syndromes.

Vaginismus, Vulvodynia, and Interstitial Cystitis

Further pelvic floor dysfunctions, which will not receive much attention in this book, include disorders such as vaginismus and vulvodynia, which are also often (but by no means always) related to psychosomatic disorders, sometimes traumatic and painful childbirth experiences, or possibly resulting from previous sexual abuse experiences. In short, vaginismus is the presence of such severe pelvic floor and vaginal muscle spasms that vaginal penetration is impossible. It can be so bad that it is even impossible to insert a tampon, a finger, etc. I recently had a patient who, after ten years of marriage, had not *once* been able to allow vaginal penetration.

Vulvodynia is a condition of intense vulvar or vaginal entrance (introitus) burning and pain, which is greatly exacerbated by contact. Again, this condition often makes sexual intercourse impossible. Recent thinking relates some cases of chronic pelvic pain, as well as cases of vulvodynia to disordered pelvic floor muscle contractions, or constant abnormal tension in the pelvic floor. Vulvodynia and interstitial cystitis (painful bladder syndrome) often occur in the same patient. Interstitial cystitis leads to severe urgency, frequency (need to go often), and severe pain when urinating, all in the absence of infection. Often, these patients get up eight to ten times a night to urinate, resulting in severe disruption of sleep quality. No wonder depression is almost universally present, which is also true in many cases of vulvodynia or other chronic pelvic pain disorders. Neither of these diseases is well understood and as a result treatment is based on flavor-of-the-month decision making. Even though well-established treatments exist for both diseases, I am not impressed by their effectiveness, underlining the fact that the etiology (cause) and pathogenesis (underlying disease process) of both conditions are poorly understood.

Psychosomatic Disorders

All humans are, to some extent, prone to psychosomatic or "somatization" disorders. These disorders occur when physical symptoms are experienced in parts of the body that are completely healthy. Possible causes could include poorly understood mechanisms whereby the brain "experiences" pain or discomfort in certain body areas, leading to behavioral changes that would presumably "protect" the individual from noxious (damaging) physical or psychological stress. These behaviors could include avoidance strategies to sex, physical activity, or work. Examples of these are common, and every physician has encountered them many times. Certainly, patients don't take kindly to being told that "it is all in your head," and this statement is not an accurate and fair description of what is actually going on. Psychosomatic disorders are extremely complex, and patients are usually not conscious of the underlying problem. Both the incidence and distribution of presentations are vastly different between the sexes. For example, in women, the pelvis is a common localization for pain and other unpleasant sensations, often with no physical "disease" as current origin.

Further complicating chronic pelvic pain is a poor understanding of the mechanisms of neural modulation and the possibility of physical changes in neural pathways as well as spinal and cortical ganglia (specialized areas of the spinal column and brain) resulting from severe physical or emotional insults to the body. What is theorized is that the severe pain or unpleasant sensations associated with pelvic infection, pregnancy complications, or even normal childbirth, could lead to physical and detectable permanent changes in the above-mentioned neural tissue, leading to future abnormal sensation of sensory stimuli from those particular body areas. Other possible causes could be severe emotional trauma during rape or sexual abuse, either current or even in the long forgotten, distant past. I'm sure I do not need to explain why psychological trauma suffered through sexual abuse would cause somatization of symptoms to the pelvic area even years later. Anyway, such neural changes could lead to chronic unpleasant sensations, or even severe pain perceived in the pelvis, even in the absence of any signs of disease by examination, or even laparoscopy. That is probably one of the common causes for negative laparoscopies in patients experiencing pelvic pain. Until very recently, our understanding of these mechanisms has been very limited, and as a result there was little that we could offer in the way of treatment, or even explanation.

One of the ways I can try to explain the phenomenon of abnormal sensation is that of ghost pain. Many who have lost limbs continue to feel their limbs very acutely. Some might even perceive them in space, even though they are not there. Pain, for instance in such a foot or hand (that doesn't exist) is common. This just shows that what causes pain in your foot, is in reality divorced from what is happening down there. It's all about the brain. The brain receives an impulse (however generated) in the "foot area" which it perceives as unpleasant—thus painful. Whether you have a foot or not is irrelevant. The same could be true for pelvic pain. Perception and reality is sometimes in conflict.

Then there is *referred* pain, the perception of pain in a body area that is completely healthy as a result of something in another body area that gives rise to painful sensations. The best known is the shoulder tip pain (usually right shoulder) that is so common after laparoscopy. What happens is that the CO_2 gas that is used to distend the abdomen irritates the phrenic nerve on the diaphragm. This nerve runs in close proximity with the nerve supplying the tip of the shoulder and has similar origins. The brain simply gets confused, like hearing a siren but not having a clue from which direction it comes.

We now know that pelvic floor biofeedback, pelvic floor strengthening exercises, and the ability to consciously relax the pelvic floor muscles could lead to improvement or even cure of many of these problems. Therefore, if your physician recommends pelvic floor physiotherapy or psychotherapy, it is not because he/she believes you are imagining things or that it is not real, but because he/she knows that it might be the ticket to a cure, or at least a way to more effectively deal with the problem.

Abdominal Wall Pain

I think it is important to discuss one other condition that often causes confusion, but which if diagnosed, can usually be effectively dealt with in short order. It never ceases to amaze me how many women referred for pelvic pain have abdominal wall pain as final diagnosis. The way to diagnose this possibility is relatively simple. If when tightening the abdominal muscles the tenderness gets worse during palpation, the origin of the tenderness is generally outside of the abdominal cavity. If the tenderness gets less, the origin is generally deeper than the muscles, thus more likely intra-abdominal in origin. Tightening of the abdominal muscles is easily accomplished by raising both legs straight, or doing a half "crunchy" (sit-up). Such tightening creates a functional "barrier," protecting the intra-abdominal contents and preventing palpation pressure from being transmitted onto these structures. Extra-abdominal abdominal wall tenderness can often be pinpointed and is often found to be acutely worse during one of these maneuvers. Treatments then would include anti-inflammatory drugs, physiotherapy, massage therapy, hot packs, or acupuncture.

Massage Therapy

Since the pelvic floor muscles can have similar trigger points of painful inflammation or spasm, the same therapies are likely to be of benefit. Massage therapy of the pelvic floor is somewhat more difficult and risqué, especially for male practitioners, but it is a technique that can lead to improvement for many women with these problems. One relatively cheap method to obtain pelvic floor massage is the utilization of certain types of vaginal vibrators, commonly found in sex stores. However, it is important to be instructed on the correct usage and models, or the results might be less than effective, even if otherwise agreeable. Women with severe vulvodynia or vaginismus might find it impossible to tolerate any kind of vaginal penetration, and treatment will obviously be different.

I cannot help but include some history here. Even though currently employed pelvic floor massage techniques have no sexual stimulation objectives, and are probably more painful than pleasurable, this has not always been the case. Unfortunately, this historical fact, as well as the sensitive nature of the treatments, makes it difficult for many women as well as most physicians to become comfortable with them.

The definition of "hysteria" was developed from the idea that most psychological, agitated states were related to the uterus ("hysteros"). It was believed that the uterus migrates around in the pelvis and abdominal cavity, creating all kinds of havoc, including "hysteria," and many other states of agitation. Treatment of these conditions involved placation of this wayward organ. This was accomplished by manual massage techniques that today could only be described as masturbation. The release of energy in the orgasmic climax was seen as the successful capture and placation of the uterus, which would then cease its disruptions, at least for a while. Until just more than a century ago, many physicians built huge practices dedicated to such treatments. Women would line up in great numbers for their "treatment" sessions, and the physicians would walk from bed to bed, performing the treatments. One practical physician saw the benefit of mechanizing the treatments to increase productivity, and it promised greatly increased income potential. This is how the vibrator was born.

Conscious Pain Mapping

Conscious pain mapping is a technique employing very small laparoscopic instruments and performing laparoscopy on a patient who is fully awake. Various areas in the abdominal and pelvic cavity are then stimulated to see if such stimulation elicits the same pain that the patient usually experiences. The idea is that one might be able to very specifically localize and pinpoint the origin of the pain, and possibly identify hidden diseases such as atypical endometriosis.

There are a few problems with the technique. Patients experience varying degrees of pain and discomfort (sometimes severe) related to the procedure. Also, the findings might be misleading. The pressure to find something is great, and patients might be cajoled subconsciously to respond in certain ways by the demeanor or assertiveness of the surgeon. There are various opinions in the gynecological literature regarding the place and usefulness of this procedure. Despite some vocal proponents, it is seldom performed. In my opinion, it is still experimental albeit a very interesting concept.

FIFTEEN
Evolution and Childbirth

My pastor once asked me whether or not I believed in evolution. This was during a general discussion of religious and denominational issues. By the way he worded this query, I suspected I was being set up—it was a test of faith, so to speak. Since I was unprepared and had not given the matter any thought for a very long time, I mumbled a somewhat incoherent response that didn't satisfy either of us. But then this question stimulated a quest for knowledge, partially to satisfy myself, but more importantly because I immediately saw the relevance of evolution to the focus of this book, namely that the development of the large human brain and skull creates significant problems during the birthing process, ones that reap certain consequences for the mother. A brief examination of anthropological and archeological findings supports this.

My research culminated in an opportunity to examine the skull of an *Australopithecus robustus* specimen as well as the pelvis and skeleton of an *Australopithecus africanus* that are estimated to be 2.5 million years old. Actually holding these skeletons in my hands was something that greatly affected my thoughts about human ancestry.

I found the 2.5-million-year-old pelvis especially interesting. That of an adult, it was quite small, but was unquestionably that of a bipedal hominid, just over four feet tall. The wide bony pelvis looked strikingly similar to that of the modern human. The pelvic inlet looked perfectly gynecoid (like that of a modern female human) with a normal pelvic inlet as well as outlet.

A few obvious facts flow from these observations. First, this individual walked upright, and probably had the same or basically the same pelvic muscle action as modern humans. Second, the shape of the pelvis suggests that the birthing process was similar to that of the modern human.

The earliest fossil records of a hominid bipedal (humanlike and walking upright) can be dated to about 3.5 million years ago. This species, called "australopithecines," had an almost human-shaped pelvis, but a much smaller brain capacity. There are numerous theories to explain the evolutionary benefit of the erect posture that ultimately contributed to the hominid species becoming the dominant species on the planet. One of the most logical theories is that by freeing the hands for purposeful manipulation of tools, the hominid gained an increased ability to defend itself and to acquire food. These factors may have led to an increased evolutionary fitness in terms of competition with other species. As a result of the increasing "free time" of the hominid arms and hands, intellectual development inevitably emerged.

Various evolutionary processes, such as the development of speech, theoretically led to a massive increase in brain capacity, sometimes to more than 67 fluid ounces (2000 ml) (the average for modern humans is on the order of 47 fluid ounces (1400 ml). This increase in brain capacity is well documented in the fossil records with a direct line that can be drawn from *Australopithecus*, through *Homo habilis* and *Homo erectus* to *Homo sapiens* (us). One viewpoint is that most, if not all, bipedal ancestral hominids were in fact, "human," with religion, speech, music, and compassion. This theory is argued using some evidence from various paleontological and archeological findings, and the presence of distinct impressions inside the skulls of some of these fossil-men, which means that they possessed the brain structures called Broca's and Wernicke's areas. These refer to the areas of the human brain essential to speech. Although new research has shown that the processing and interpretation of speech occurs much more widespread throughout the brain than previously believed, these two areas are definitely crucial. If one accepts that most of these fossil-men had spoken language, religion, compassion, and made music, the only logical deduction is that they were self-conscious beings and in a certain sense at least could be considered "human," however primitive. The term "human" is however surprisingly problematic. We are so used to seeing ourselves in total isolation from the rest of nature that a glimpse of our real place in nature comes as a revelation (not necessarily a pleasant one).

With the benefits of bipedalism (walking upright on two legs) came certain problems. An upright stance created the all-too-common problem of lower back pain. Another problem was the size, structure, and function of the pelvis. A balance had to be found between a more efficient, thus narrower pelvis (the faster you could run, the more likely you were to survive) and a pelvis of adequate size to allow birth of a big-brained infant with a larger head. This point is well illustrated by comparing the increased efficiency of the various muscles implanted in the male pelvis in comparison to the female pelvis. This balance between efficiency and adequacy was a critical development in human evolution and led to what I would call the "mechanical imperative." The pelvic structures suddenly became the main support of the body cavity. This development brought tremendous challenges, some of which, it is fair to say, have not been totally solved.

When we look at the animal kingdom, we find that in most mammals the pelvic "floor" is not a floor at all, but a wall. Since the usual primate posture for the body is mostly horizontal, the brunt of the intra-abdominal weight does not continuously fall on this structure, but rather onto the anterior abdominal wall and the pubic bone. In the human, the pelvic floor became the most important support structure for the pelvic and abdominal contents. The pelvic floor counteracts the full force of gravity; and with weak pelvic floor muscles, the fascial layers are the last defense against prolapse.

In nature's scheme of things, the integrity of the pelvic floor over time is, after all, not all that important. By the time pelvic floor disorders become significant problems the most important biological functions, which ensure the survival of our species (namely, reproduction), have been completed. Furthermore, since these disorders usually lead to a personal loss of quality of life rather than decreased life expectancy, they have had no discernable influence on the course of evolutionary development. For most of human history, people rarely survived to an age where it did become a problem. Fortunately, people today live much longer. So it is imperative for us to look at the pelvic floor with new eyes, and to develop new strategies to protect it from time and aging.

We will now take a simplified tour through the evolutionary development of the pelvis, which will illustrate how this area of the body has changed and adapted to the altered life circumstances of our ancestors.

According to evolutionary theory, life developed in marine waters, in surroundings where the specific gravity of the aqueous environment was the same as that of the body of the organisms and they could thus be considered weightless. Only rudimentary support systems were required to keep their bodies together. In fish for instance, the pelvis is very rudimentary, has no support function at all, and no sphincter muscles are present. The first vertebrates that moved onto land were amphibians; and for the first time, some support function became necessary for the pelvis, to counteract gravity. The development of air breathing required the development of a ribcage and abdominal muscles, which also led to an increased pressure gradient in the body cavity that had to be countered by an increasingly sophisticated pelvic floor, although there are still no sphincter muscles.

The first vertebrates that completely escaped the bondage of the marine environment were reptiles. This extraordinary development led to a virtual explosion of evolutionary experimentation, and the success of all the dinosaurs and other prehistoric animals that so occupy our imagination.

Even in dinosaurs it is easy to see how bipedalism affected the pelvic girdle. The pelvis of the quadruped dinosaurs differs completely from the biped ones, with evidence of a support function developing in the biped ones. Of course the dinosaurs were ultimately doomed, but their reign had a great influence on the evolution of mammalian animals. Some theories suggest that placental reproduction developed in part as a result of the need for a longer intra-uterine developmental process, in order for the newborn mammalian to be able to retreat from the incredible dangerous world it was born into. The mammalian body cavity developed the two-compartment system by development of a thoracic diaphragm, in order to be able to create a higher intra-abdominal and intrathoracic pressure, which helps with tissue oxygenation (oxygen uptake). This development was required by the need to develop more efficient muscle systems, quicker reflexes, and faster running speeds, as a result of the dangers, and the increasing competition of the world they found themselves in. This higher-pressure system brought new challenges to the pelvic area where efficient methods to control the excretory systems and openings had to be found. To solve these problems, the development of the various pelvic bones and systems can be followed through the animal kingdom, from prehistoric to contemporary. Differences between animal types become quite obvious and are understandable in light of their widely different lifestyles. Most pronograde (quadruped) animals like dogs don't have a significant problem with pressure in the pelvis, except when leaping or jumping. Under these circumstances the tail is pulled in tightly against the perineum to help close off the perineal (pelvic) opening. Many carnivorous mammalians have developed strong sphincter muscles, strong pelvic floor muscles (levator muscles), and a strong tail-closing mechanism. By contrast, in herbivorous animals these muscles are much weaker. The reason is obvious. The lifestyle of carnivorous animals leads to the generation of much higher intra-abdominal pressures, and the need for the pelvic outlet to be able to counteract this.

In primates, with the assumption of an upright bipedal position, the pelvic floor muscles become the primary supports for the intra-abdominal organs. This is a result of the fact that the pubic symphysis becomes part of the abdominal wall, and thus loses any possible direct support function. The perineal tail closure mechanism disappears, with only the coccygeal segments (coccyx—the very tip of the spinal canal that can be felt right at the beginning of the buttock cleft) remaining as a strong but flexible anchoring point for many of the pelvic floor muscles and sphincters. A further development was the replacements of some muscles with fascia, ligaments, and tendons (refer to chapter 3).

Further adaptations that help to protect the human pelvic floor from pressure from above, include the progressive skeletal changes that occur in the maturation of the spinal skeleton from childhood to adulthood. In the young child, the spine is almost straight and the pelvic cavity is small. Too small in fact, to accommodate the organs that are considered "pelvic" organs in the adult. These organs thus lie mostly in the abdominal cavity. With increasing pressure on the back of the pelvis as the child grows, especially after the normal human erect posture is attained, the pelvic cavity changes in shape to become the hollow cavity of the adult. The reason is the constant pressure from above, mostly directed posteriorly (backward) and inferiorly (downward) toward and into the sacral bone. On the other hand, the muscles implanted on it are pulling the tip of the sacrum forward. Over time, the sacrum inevitably changes shape to the curved structure we know, only attaining equilibrium when final ossification of the skeleton (late puberty) precludes any further shape changes. One positive result of this change in shape and position of the pelvic cavity is the fact that at least part of it became protected from direct forces from above, by the hollow of the sacrum, and the promontory of the sacrum (the prominent ridge formed by the junction of the spine and the sacrum).

After the evolutionary disappearance of the tail, the strength and thickness of the posterior (back) parts of the levator ani muscles decreased significantly. Much of these muscles changed into fibrous tissue, with the result that mostly the anterior (forward), and lateral (side) parts of the levator ani persisted as muscle tissue. A further result of the developing orthograde (erect) position was a forward shift of the visceral canals (organs that protrude the pelvic floor, namely the urethra, vagina, and recto-anum). This shift led to their increased exposure to pressure gradients from above, and compensatory hypertrophy of the levator ani muscles in this area. In humans, the puborectalis muscle thus became extremely important, as well as the strongest part of the levator ani. This muscle is further described in the section on the anatomy of the pelvic floor. Further mechanisms to compensate for the tendency for visceral protrusion involve the provision of relatively strong sphincter mechanisms that not only close off the hollow organ tubes, but also help with support, as a result of their common origin from parts of the levator ani muscles, and attachments to strong points such as the perineal body and coccygeal ligaments as mentioned above.

One theory that tries to explain the increased evolutionary fitness of *Homo sapiens* is the development of speech, which made communication and the development of culture possible. Hence the onset of the exceptionally large human brain, the main reason for our tremendous success as a species. However, our large brains come with a price.

As stated, the large human brain and skull creates significant problems for the birthing process. Certainly the fetus survives best if it is large, but this has obvious consequences for the mother. The birthing process can be likened to a competitive interaction between the mother and her fetus, with some common ideals (such as the survival of both), but also some divergent goals, namely to personally emerge from the experience in as good a shape as possible.

Recent evidence from scientific studies has indicated the possibility that the pregnant mother can directly influence the size of her unborn fetus, especially toward the end of her pregnancy. It has been shown that this observation holds true even in the setting of donor embryos from larger genetic parents into smaller surrogate mothers, who deliver smaller infants than might have been suspected. The theoretical way the birth mother can accomplish this is by restricting the blood flow to her uterus, thereby affecting the availability of nutrients to the fetus.

This finding may be evidence of the mother's attempt to protect her own interests to the general detriment of the fetus. Of course it should be self-evident that if there were an insurmountable discrepancy between the pelvis of the mother and the size of the fetus, it would also pose a clear disadvantage for the infant. This "mechanical imperative" may explain the relative underdevelopment (altriciality) of the human newborn infant compared to most other primates. Gestational restriction (that is, restriction of time for growth) is another evolutionary development to permit human birth. The human newborn has been called an "extragestational fetus," which means that it still has fetal qualities but now has to survive outside the uterus. It also implies that, if not for the mechanical pelvic "imperative," human gestation might have been much longer. This comparative underdevelopment of the human newborn obviously required the development of strong social groups to share the tasks necessary for survival. This absolute requirement to the success (so far) of our species could have been the main stimulus for the development of culture. We are truly locked into a cooperative struggle against the forces of nature and evolution. No man (or woman) is an island.

Certain theoretical advantages have been attributed to this "premature" birth of the human fetus. In comparison to other primate species, for instance gorillas and chimpanzees, the human newborn's brain, although bigger, is less developed in relation to the final adult brain. Now, everybody knows that the first few years of a child's life are critical for the formation not only of personality, but also of brain development and intelligence. The human infant, because of its early birth, is exposed to and bombarded with all the stimuli and brain-forming sensory inputs that its now "extrauterine" world provides. By contrast, at a similar developmental level, the small gorilla and chimpanzee fetus, sensory deprived, is still wallowing in its amniotic fluid while its brain develops further with only genetic input.

One further ingenious development in the human birth process was the advent of the rotation of the fetus as it moves down the birth canal. At any given time the longest axis of the presenting part of the fetus (usually the head) has to fit in the corresponding axis of the pelvis. Since the human female pelvis is widest transversely (side to side) at the entrance and widest longitudinally (front to back) at the exit, the fetus *has* to rotate. Nonrotation is a common reason for failure to progress in labor and the subsequent emergency cesarean. There is some debate about whether this feature, which is a characteristic and essential element of human birth, was also present in fossil-man (or rather woman). I believe that it was.

Evolutionary theory purports that "reproductively unfit" mothers, with pelvises too small to give birth, would die during childbirth and thus not propagate their (or their partner's) genes. The baby would almost always die as well. The other side of the coin is that the inability of those babies with increasing brain size to be born alive theoretically inhibited any further evolutionary brain size development.

Our ability to deliver babies safely by cesarean section in cases of obstructed labor has revolutionized our ability to intervene in nature. This ability has not only removed the necessity for an adequate pelvis, but also the impediment to possible further evolutionary brain-size development.

The question has been asked whether evolution, as a species shaping force, is still active in humans. As a result of our intellectual ability to subject nature to our collective will, many of the selection pressures of the Darwinian model aren't valid in our species anymore. By safely delivering and helping babies who would otherwise have died, we have escaped the tyranny of raw natural selection. This is not only the result of modern medicine of course. Our whole society has a role to play here.

Whether selection still plays a subtle role in the human race, however, is an interesting question with no definite answer, as further details as to how evolution precisely operates are still being examined.

SIXTEEN
The Complexity of Choice

"Last year, I requested five times to have a cesarean section," says Angela, a thirty-three-year-old financial consultant. "My husband and I were told that there were no risks to me to deliver vaginally because my baby was not breech or over ten pounds. I was told I was being paranoid and unrealistic to think that a cesarean section would be a better choice for me. Sadly, they were wrong and now I have learned so much about the problems I never knew so many women are dealing with. Six months after my delivery, my cervix is an inch from coming out of my vagina. The protrusions into my vagina make intercourse impossible. In addition, I have stress incontinence. I have not resumed my career as I am hoping to have surgery in the next year. My physical, mental, emotional, marital, and financial status has been rocked by this unfortunate event. Last year, my gut was telling me what was right for me, but no one would respect my wishes, or even give me a truthful answer about the risks. When a professional woman in the prime of her life cannot make choices about her body, there is definitely something wrong."

✣ ✣ ✣

This book supports the concept that a woman should have the right to choose how her baby is to be delivered, whether vaginally or via an elective cesarean section. It does *not* argue that *all* women should have a cesarean section. In many cases, the risks of cesarean birth will outweigh the benefits, and a vaginal delivery will *clearly* be preferable. There is a very clear distinction between elective cesarean section, chosen by the well-informed woman in consultation with her physician, and any unwanted and unnecessary cesarean sections that are thrust upon the woman who desires a vaginal birth.

In 1914, the U.S. Supreme Court formalized into law the concept of autonomous patient choice. The law stated that every adult human being has the right to determine what should be done with one's own body, and that no surgeon could perform an operation without the patient's consent. From that, in the 1950s, the practice of *informed* consent developed. After a medical diagnosis is made, and treatment options and risks are fully disclosed, the patient has the right to choose from the given alternatives.

But the concept of autonomous choice and informed consent is not as straightforward where pregnancy is concerned. Much has been written about this issue in medical journals of late, but little discussion on this topic is reaching the general public—until now.

Lisa H. Harris, M.D., covered the issue in her journal article entitled "Counseling Women About Choice."[1] We will refer to this work throughout this chapter. She wrote:

> Decisions concerning route of delivery in pregnancy are distinctly different, however, from decisions outside of pregnancy for two important reasons. The most obvious, of course, is the presence of the fetus. How and to what degree fetal interests are to be considered in decisions about cesarean is not a straightforward issue. Consent for delivery is also different from consent in other medical arenas because labor and delivery are unlike other "medical" events—they are inevitable physiological processes. "Choosing" vaginal delivery is usually not a choice at all; it will occur unless a surgical intervention is made prior.

Later in the article she writes:

> In most areas of medicine, when a variety of alternatives are available to achieve an outcome, patients are offered a choice, even if one alternative carries more risk but has benefits valued highly by the patient. This has not been the case for route of delivery. A 1986 survey of physicians showed that 92–95% of physicians would not perform a cesarean in the absence of conventional indication. Why are women not offered a choice of delivery route? As one author writing in this area asks, "In this era of patient choice, should information regarding potential benefits of elective cesarean delivery be given to women?"

Harris also cites an editorial submitted by W. Benson Harer, a past president of the American College of Obstetricians and Gynecologists (ACOG). He expresses his views and not necessarily those of ACOG. Harer states that paternalism is at stake in this debate. Paternalism means treating a patient as if she is incapable of exercising responsible choice . . . free choice of route of delivery belongs on the list of women's civil and reproductive rights that already includes property rights, education, voting, contraception, and abortion. Why must route of delivery be dictated to women by the medical profession?

At the 2001 meeting of the Society of Obstetricians and Gynecologists of Canada (SOCG), 62 percent of the gynecologists and family physicians present voted that they are in favor of increased autonomy in the choice of delivery route, and that elective cesarean section should be a viable option.

Physicians have a duty to supply patients with the information necessary to make informed decisions regarding their medical care. Often, women do not have the amount or kind of information that allows active participation in the decision-making process regarding labor and delivery. The correlation between vaginal birth and severe pelvic floor damage is rarely discussed or viewed as a compulsory part of routine prenatal *care.*

Again Harris cites several studies showing that regardless of whether surgery was elective or emergent, when women felt involved in the decision early on, nearly all were satisfied with their procedure. When women did not feel involved in the decision, almost one-third felt dissatisfied with the surgical process.

It is very important to note that a recent survey in the United Kingdom found that one-third of all female obstetricians polled indicated that they would choose elective cesarean birth, given the choice. Their reasoning indicated the specific protection of the pelvic floor. Eighty percent of those who indicated a preference for an elective cesarean birth cited the fear of long-term consequences associated with vaginal birth. The main consequences feared included stress urinary incontinence and anal fecal incontinence. Further concerns included the effects of vaginal birth on their future sexuality and sexual function. A minority of these professional women stressed the concern for fetal health as a main reason for elective cesarean birth. Similar results were obtained during informal surveys in Canada.

The telling responses of these knowledgeable women are solid proof that a serious debate is overdue. If female obstetricians feel so strongly about the potential long-term negative effects of vaginal birth that they would increasingly choose elective cesarean births for themselves, then the question needs to be asked: What are physicians telling their patients? Do they discuss the risks of vaginal birth with their patients? Perhaps they do not. Due to the medicopolitical and health care–economic climate in most Western countries today, patients are being denied knowledge and opportunities to make important health care choices.

It is hoped that in the future, women will have increased opportunities to make decisions regarding childbirth based upon what is important to them as individuals. This will involve constant interaction with the cultural, political, and economic agendas of the day.

Many will argue that women are making their own decisions, and that this entire debate is really a nonissue outside the medical community. However, does every woman have adequate information upon which to base a decision? Arguably, it is time that facts about the pelvic floor are introduced into the equation. Not as a scare tactic, but as a useful contribution to the debate on this long-overdue issue surrounding women's health.

The Politics of Childbirth

Childbirth is such a fundamental and integral part of the human experience that its potential to create conflict is not surprising. Throughout the ages, the policies and practices of childbirth closely reflect the given historical, cultural, and political ethos.

During the twentieth century, the medical revolution changed not only the way we bring babies into the world, but also the very process of conception. These changes were, to a large degree, the result of key medical breakthroughs such as the discovery of microorganisms, antibiotics, and improved fetal monitoring. The development of ways to monitor the intra-uterine fetus brought about revolutionary change (some of which, as discussed later in chapter 17, actually prompts unnecessary intervention). Conflicts arose between the well-being of the fetus versus that of the mother. Previously, interference for the fetus's sake posed such a hazard to maternal well-being that the fetus was relegated to secondary status as nature was left to take its course, with often fatal consequences for the fetus. The improved operative vaginal delivery procedures, antibiotics, and more aseptic technique provided, for the first time, the ability to safely intervene to expedite delivery in some cases. The development of anesthetics and innovative surgical techniques, coupled with potent antibiotics, took obstetrics to a new level. Suddenly it was possible to deliver fetuses prior to the commencement of or at the very early stage of labor. As cesarean sections became safer and more standardized, the beneficial effects on labor outcome in many cases led to increased usage, even to the point where it was sometimes done unnecessarily.

The above changes coincided with a cultural revolution of numbing proportions. Whereas women usually delivered at home, attended by family members or a midwife, they now started to deliver in hospitals and clinics, and were attended by doctors or highly qualified nurses and midwives. Then in most of the Western world the midwife gave way to the family practitioner or specialist obstetrician. The homelike atmosphere of the childbirth experience changed into a full-blown "medical" event, with intravenous infusions, monitors, sterile packs, artificial bright lights, gowned physicians, and restrictions on who might attend. The decision to perform invasive procedures became the sole responsibility of the attending physician. Cesarean sections were sometimes performed increasingly for dubious indications, which led to an inevitable and incredible rise in operative delivery rates.

The aforementioned changes were coincident with dramatic falls in both maternal and perinatal mortality (deaths of mothers and newborn babies) and morbidity (complications). One could be excused for the assumption that everyone would be happy—but not so. The advent of such rapid change and the often-perceived dehumanizing face of modern obstetrics ensured that a backlash was not long in coming.

Referring once again to the Harris article, she writes:

> History provides some insight into why choice around cesarean on demand is complex. We have faced remarkably similar moments in obstetrical history before—moments in which it was unclear whether women's choices were liberating or ultimately further disempowering. Changes in childbirth in the 19th century saw female-dominated midwifery give way to male-dominated, technologically oriented obstetrical professionalism. . . . This period is often depicted as the height of paternalism in care of birthing women.

Harris then points to the respected writings of Judith Walzer Leavitt, author of the book *Brought to Bed*, a look at childbirth history from 1750 to 1950. This book is often a popular choice by major universities in the women's health studies curriculum. Harris notes that Leavitt insightfully showed that medical paternalism is more complex than it appears on its face. Leavitt's research showed that women were not passive victims of male medical interventions, but that women welcomed interventions that made labor appear to be less painful and safer. Harris interjects, though, that labor did not necessarily become safer in early hospital care, as physicians were responsible for hundreds of deaths from puerperal sepsis. But she writes that Leavitt was one of the first historians to make the very important observation that women's choices in childbirth are complex. Harris further states:

> a historical tension around women's choice exists. Our contemporary debate over cesarean on demand reflects these same tensions—women are active agents, seeking relief from fears of labor and debility, but what is demanded from medicine, and what medicine can offer, may ultimately disempower women. Although history does not provide an answer for our contemporary crossroads around cesarean, it does remind us that we have been here before, and probably will again, as childbirth technologies continue to flourish.

To some, these concepts might seem to inspire a paralysis over choice, a quandary of self-doubt. A mantra in one's head might chant incessantly, "Am I right? Am I wrong? Am I right? Am I wrong?" So much so that one might simply rely upon what *feels* right. And although there is definitely a great deal to be said about women's intuition, there may be little value in relying solely on gut instinct when real empowerment arguably lies with information and education. Information is power. There is a dearth of information readily available. With that said, there is no doubt that we can become empowered by informed choice.

The difficulty lies in the politics of choice. One group lobbies for this, another for that. They may seem to have such divergent opinions that obviously somebody has to be right and somebody has to be wrong. Who do you believe? This is where your gut and your spirit do help you to make a choice. Because you have to choose what *you* feel is right for *you,* after weighing all the information and all the risks of either decision. If you have truly done that, then *whatever* choice you make is truly the *right* choice.

Choice in a Competitive Environment

My initial experience with obstetrics as a medical student in South Africa was under the direct supervision of nurse-midwives. I respected the fact that they knew infinitely more about normal labors than I did at that time. I respect them and their function in the system, but feel that the current competitive environment that has developed between midwives and obstetricians is quite unfortunate. The current political system in obstetrical care in western Canada forces midwives to do home deliveries, a policy that I strongly disagree with. To me, it would be much preferable if midwives and physicians could work together in an integrated system.

Today, most maternity units try to create a more homelike atmosphere. Not that long ago, fathers played a peripheral role in the childbirth process, whereas now they are welcomed and encouraged to be integrally involved throughout the experience. Today's women read multiple books on labor and delivery, and they work out birthing plans, which are then presented to their obstetrician or midwife. This sometimes irritates obstetricians greatly, and a few bemoan the loss of their hitherto unchallenged professional autonomy. And some midwives promote the birthing plan as a way to avoid the "evils" of medical intervention.

The Associated Press reports that more than 4,000 practicing nurse-midwives attended 185,000 births in the United States in 1992, or almost 5 percent of the total. Of those 185,000 births, 95 percent were in hospitals. In the early 1900s, midwives attended 40 percent of all births in the United States, but their role diminished as obstetricians and other doctors took over deliveries, a trend that obviously resulted in much ill will between midwives and physicians.

In an article written by Faith Gibson, a certified professional midwife (CPM), the decline of midwifery is described as "the hundred year's war against midwives." Gibson maintains that influential medical politicians embarked on a well-documented, well-coordinated, and well-financed strategy to eliminate the midwife from the practice of her own profession. And indeed, the profession is being challenged. In some states, statutes require midwives to have nursing degrees in order to practice, while in others, licensure is unavailable, indirectly preventing midwives from practicing legally.

Midwife Adrian E. Feldhusen writes that, ". . . in the early 1970s, women's groups encouraged a revival of lay midwifery. Feminists argued that medical care needed to be demystified and women's lives demedicalized. They maintained that childbirth is not a disease and that normal deliveries do not require hospitalization and the supervision of an obstetrician. Soon the conflict over homebirth proved to be one of the most bitter between the medical profession and the women's movement. While no state forbade homebirth, the American College of Obstetricians and Gynecologists (ACOG) actively discouraged it."[2]

But today, feminist attitudes toward cesarean sections have shifted, largely from natural childbirth to choice. Feminist editorial is supporting the concept that women should have autonomy over decisions affecting their bodies. For example, some feminists say, if a woman wants to have an epidural, or another C-section rather than risk uterine rupture, it should be up to her. As such, while 5 percent of pregnant women find homebirth the preferable choice, the majority opts for the hospital environment.

Online reports from *NurseWeek* indicate that ACOG has issued several statements *implying* that labor and delivery are hazardous events and therefore require "standards of safety which are provided in the hospital setting and cannot be matched in the home situation." *NurseWeek* also cites a joint statement between the American College of Nurse-Midwives (ACNM) and ACOG that says that the ideal model of practice is where a qualified obstetrician/gynecologist directs the maternity care team.

One inevitable result of the climate of guilt that the natural childbirth enthusiasts promote is the feeling of failure in those women who do not successfully deliver their babies vaginally without instrumentation or at all. Not only is this a likely explanation for the recognized higher incidence of postpartum depression in woman undergoing cesarean section (discussed in more detail below), but also it can potentially interfere with the new mother's bonding with her newborn baby.

In the study entitled, "Psychological Aspects of Cesarean Section," its author, Sarah Clement, Ph.D., covers the importance of cultural attitudes and their effects upon childbearing women. Her research points to an obvious implication that in populations that *do not* adhere to the "natural birth culture," cesarean birth is experienced very positively. The opposite would be true in those cultures *with* a "natural" model. For instance, the Brazilian culture *values* the cesarean birth as it is thought to symbolize modernity and technology.

I certainly do not oppose the goal of a vaginal delivery that requires no intervention. This is a very laudable and positive accomplishment. My problem is with the concept (currently being promoted by various groups) that intervention during childbirth is almost *always* unnecessary, unnatural, and detrimental. Much has been made in the media, as well as in certain publications and books, about the fact that specialist obstetricians have a higher intervention rate than midwives. Lobby groups pushing their agendas, in this case the minimalist approach, use this. To my mind, this is similar to stating that a corporal does a better job than a general, because the general's decisions will probably lead to a higher loss of equipment and personnel in battle. Of course the obstetrician will have a higher intervention rate. He or she is, after all, trained to do just that, and do it safely too. Obstetricians will naturally receive most of the complicated cases that require intervention, even if the patients started off as low-risk, primary care cases. With statistics thus skewed, one can easily seem to prove any point.

We'd all like to think that medical professionals and their patients could put aside their differences and work as the perfect team, but in our *imperfect* world, that doesn't always happen. We can strive though for a healthy debate, and in the process, we can learn something from one another. Certainly this competitive environment makes it far more difficult for women to choose between homebirth or the hospital, midwife or obstetrician, and vaginal or cesarean birth. After all, both sides may seem to be just as rigid, and just as passionate about the way things should be done. Again this is why information, education, and proactive *individual* choice are so important.

The Psychology of Choice and Cesarean Birth

Although there are a number of studies that have looked at the differences in psychological outcome between women who have had vaginal deliveries and those who have had cesarean deliveries, none of them really answer the question that is pertinent for us, namely: Would there be a difference between women undergoing chosen elective cesarean birth versus chosen vaginal birth? Most of the studies so far have compared women who have had vaginal delivery to women who have had cesareans—period. The problem with this biased assessment should be immediately obvious. Certainly, the overwhelming majority of women who ended up undergoing a cesarean section had it as an emergency procedure, whereas they had preferred to have a natural vaginal delivery.

It is obvious that an emergency procedure and an emergency cesarean section even more so, is a very traumatic event and is often associated with great fear, not only for the sake of the baby, but also for oneself. Especially in an emergency situation, the real or perceived lack of control over one's destiny can inspire a significantly negative reaction. Usually this negative reaction is short-lived, especially if the outcome is a happy one. Sometimes however, the feeling of loss of control can be long lasting and intense. It could lead to problems bonding with the baby and problems in the relationship with the spouse. This is, of course, because an emergency cesarean is by definition a procedure that is done when things have gone wrong, or at least not as desired or expected. It is therefore not surprising to find that cesarean birth could be viewed as a less satisfactory childbirth experience when compared with vaginal birth, at least in the studies presented in the literature. Women who had emergency cesarean sections under general anesthesia were the least satisfied. Frequently mentioned reasons for dissatisfaction were the expressed disappointment of "not being there" for the birth of their baby. Even so, there is no unanimity in this, and numerous articles have shown no significant difference.

I would accept, however, that there are real differences between these two groups in satisfaction rates. This is one of the reasons I am in support of following strict guidelines before recommending cesarean sections for women who want to experience a vaginal delivery.

I strongly believe—and there is some evidence to support this view—that women who choose elective cesarean sections are much more satisfied than those who experience a cesarean on an emergency basis. In fact, it seems that there is very little difference in satisfaction between the vaginal birth group and women who choose elective cesarean section. For these women, cesarean is not seen as a *failure.* Importantly, they did not suffer through the emotional ups and downs of a long and complicated labor, which was ultimately unsuccessful. They were well rested, well hydrated, and knew exactly when their babies would be born. They knew what to expect and had the support of a spouse who also knew what to expect, and who could therefore be of emotional support.

Elective cesarean sections are almost never performed under general anesthetic, thus the entry of the newborn baby into the world is experienced as an immediate, personal, and joint occasion by the couple. These women overwhelmingly feel empowered by the fact that they had significant input into the decision, and that ultimately it is their personal choice.

In Support of Choice

In the last few years, *American Medical News* has issued reports regarding a woman's right to choose. *AM News* staff reporter Deborah Shelton noted comments from several of today's medical experts currently speaking out on the topic. David Campbell Walters, M.D., is in private practice in Mount Vernon, Illinois. He is the author of the book *Just Take It Out! The Ethics and Economics of Cesarean Sections and Hysterectomy.* Walters says to *AM News,* "It is well established that autonomy is the governing principle in medicine, at least for a woman wishing to refuse a cesarean delivery. And yet, while the vast majority of obstetricians would respect a woman's right to refuse a cesarean delivery, nobody is interested in respecting a woman's desire to refuse a vaginal birth. What we are actually choosing between is either elective cesarean delivery or attempted vaginal birth, followed by emergency cesarean delivery, *if* vaginal birth fails. Recent literature shows that emergency cesarean deliveries are at least twice as dangerous as elective ones are. This is important if we are going to look at the ethics of how we are going to manage our patients."

AM News also quoted from an editorial written by W. Benson Harer, M.D. Harer wrote in an ACOG publication:

> Women are often bullied into having a vaginal birth even when they are appropriate candidates for elective cesarean delivery. Patients should be given information about their individual situations—what the risks and benefits are for vaginal delivery vs. cesarean delivery—and then be allowed to make their own choices in conjunction with their physician. It's a matter of informed consent. The continual advances of anesthesia, asepsis, neonatal care, and surgical techniques have reduced the risks of cesarean delivery. Perhaps the time has come when the risks, benefits, and costs are so balanced between cesarean and vaginal delivery that the deciding factor should simply be the mother's preference for how her baby is to be delivered.[3]

Partners in Informed Choice

Sara Paterson-Brown is a consultant in obstetrics and gynecology in the United Kingdom. Her articles on choice are readily available on the Internet. Paterson feels that doctors should perform an elective cesarean section upon request as long as the woman is fully informed. She stresses that *this does not mean that obstetricians should become technicians at the mercy of women's choice, but that they should be partners in the process of decision making*. Women should have a pivotal role in their obstetric care, she says, "yet some are now being criticized for the choices they are making. These choices should not be discredited simply because they are not the ones that were expected. We should respect a woman's view and choice if it is fully informed, if she expresses a logical reason for wanting a cesarean section, and if she can demonstrate an understanding of the implications of the procedure. We should not be dictating to women what they should think, nor should we be judgmental of their values if they happen to differ from our own."

It may be time now to replace "natural" and "normal" in the practice in midwifery and obstetrics with "an open concept of the good." If this approach is adopted it will not be the professionals who will decide what is good and what is bad, but instead the informed and autonomous woman in pregnancy.[4]

Notes

1. Lisa H. Harris, "Counseling Women About Choice," *Best Practice and Research Clinical Obstetrics and Gynaecology* 15, no. 1 (2001): 100–103.
2. Adrian E. Feldhusen, "The History of Midwifery and Childbirth in America: A Timeline," *Midwifery Today* (2000).
3. W. Benson Harer, "Patient Choice Cesarean," *ACOG Clinical Review* 5, no. 2 (2000): 13–16.
4. Michael Stephen Robson, "Can We Reduce the Cesarean Rate?" *Best Practice and Research Clinical Obstetrics and Gynaecology* 15, no. 1 (2001): 190.

SEVENTEEN
The Great Cesarean Rate Debate

Change is inevitable, and it is well known that change often brings conflict. Family practitioners, obstetricians, and midwives often pit themselves against one another with conflicting interests. Government and health maintenance organizations (HMOs) are increasingly involved in the active management of health care and maternity care. Not only do they often develop different fee schedules, but they also actively encourage and often force patients into specific channels or modes of care. The reduction of cesarean birth rates is very high on their agenda.

Their involvement should be viewed with suspicion, as their main interest is most certainly an economic one. Government studies usually focus on population outcomes and global costs. After all, for governments, the individual patient's situation does not hold much importance in the global scheme of things. Likewise, costs that might be incurred many years down the line are not considered. Instead, with their short-term thinking they consider only the direct costs of vaginal versus cesarean birth, and vaginal birth is clearly the cheaper of the two.

Yet there are more than four hundred thousand operations per year in the United States for genital prolapse alone, most of which can be directly related to vaginal childbirth. This number is certainly likely to take a significant leap in the very near future as the baby boomer generation ages. No study that we have found has ever taken the cost of genital prolapse surgery into consideration when compiling cost differences between vaginal and cesarean birth. Loss of economic activity and productivity in those who are seriously affected by pelvic floor damage, and in those who are recovering from corrective surgery are also not considered.

Determining the "correct" cesarean rate has been an ongoing debate for the past twenty-five years. From 1970 to 1999, the rate of cesarean delivery in the United States rose from 5 percent to 23 percent, with a peak of 25 percent in 1988. There is a significant pressure, particularly (and not surprisingly) from governmental agencies and insurance providers, to lower the current rate, as it is felt to be at an unacceptable level and resulting from unacceptable indications. Arguably, the cesarean rate is a loaded issue with many factions weighing in, each with perhaps a different motivation. This debate dramatically affects the complexity behind the concept of patient choice and elective cesarean section.

In response to the rising cesarean section rate, the U.S. Department of Health and Human Services initiated an agenda in 1987 (called Healthy People 2000) to lower the cesarean rate to 15 percent by the year 2000, a goal that has not been met. It was not a mandate, the department says, but a guide toward reaching what *they feel* is a desirable rate. How this number was arrived at has never been made clear. Nevertheless, the insurance industry jumped on the bandwagon to declare a 15 percent target rate as *the* number by which all are judged. They say that the motivation is to increase lifespan, add preventative services, and reduce discrepancies in health care among U.S. citizens. But the motivation is undoubtedly an economic one. With cesarean birth running an extra $3,000 in surgical costs per delivery, the estimated savings by reaching the target rate were $1 billion annually. Consider that the U.S. government is the largest purchaser of health insurance, while the insurance lobbyists are incredibly powerful entities. To increase profits, they must cut costs, but they certainly don't pass any of those savings on to the consumer. Have you ever experienced a decrease in your premiums? Do you easily attain every payment that you think they should make? Can one ever truly understand what an insurance policy says? Across the board, the answer is no—and there is a reason for that.

Admirably, in 1999, four Boston obstetricians took a stand against the rate debate in an article in the *New England Journal of Medicine*. As there is no evidence to support this target rate, the authors declare it as being economically motivated, and most importantly state that, "it may have a detrimental effect on maternal and infant health." Essentially, they question just who is calling the shots in health care. Setting a target rate is an authoritarian approach to health care delivery, they say. It implies that women should have no say in their own care. The risks and benefits of various approaches clearly need to be discussed with patients. The National Health Service in the United Kingdom has taken the approach that consumers' choices must be considered; we should do the same.[1]

In the same vein, participants at the 2001 ACOG annual meeting expressed that a cesarean target rate has long been used as a pressure tactic and a "quality measurement" by insurers and managed care organizations, but that ultimately a cesarean delivery should be based on patient choice and individual physiology and circumstances.

As stated in the May 2001 issue of *American Medical News*, the pressure to reduce the cesarean rates comes primarily because the procedure is viewed as more expensive and involves longer hospital stays. According to data presented by Dr. Linda Brubaker, professor of obstetrics and gynecology at Loyola Medical Center, the morbidity (complications) and expenses associated with C-sections would be viewed as lower if vaginal birth-related pelvic floor injuries were considered in the picture. Brubaker says, "We need to resist the financial quotas that managed care companies are putting on us and encourage them to broaden their window to look at the entire woman's lifespan, and include pelvic floor complications and the cost of its treatment in their financial analysis."

Reasons for Cesarean Increase

Obstetricians acknowledge that a decline in vaginal births among women with previous cesarean sections is one major reason for the recent surge. Medical studies also list a variety of other factors behind the rise in cesarean sections. They may include an increasing climate of medical litigation, the prevalence of electronic fetal monitoring (EFM) with its high false-positive rate, the increased use of epidural anesthesia, and inherent time management problems developed within the medical system. Importantly, the rise in maternal age as well as the improved safety of cesarean deliveries has also had a significant effect. Some of these issues and others demand a closer look.

Vaginal Birth After Cesarean Delivery

It is now accepted that vaginal delivery after one or even two previous cesareans is possible and is likely to be successful. However, there are risks that should be addressed before a patient can make a fully informed decision. ACOG states that most patients who have had a low-transverse uterine incision from a previous cesarean delivery and who have no contraindications for vaginal birth are candidates for a trial of labor. Women who have had two previous low-transverse cesarean deliveries also may be considered for a vaginal birth, but the risk of uterine rupture increases with the number of previous uterine incisions. ACOG recommends that women with a classical (vertical) scar have a repeat cesarean birth. A rupture for this type of scar has been reported between 4 and 9 percent. The classical scar is on the higher, thicker, and more muscular part of the uterus. Because this is the part of the uterus that generates the most force, a scar in this area can lead to an explosive "blowout" rupture.

Once again, vaginal birth after previous cesarean (VBAC) is a hot topic. Over the last decade, the attitude toward VBAC had changed from "once a cesarean always a cesarean" to, in effect, "once a cesarean always a VBAC attempt."

Studies report that the VBAC rate in the United States increased from 3.5 percent in 1980 to almost 25 percent by 1993, meaning that almost half of all pregnant women with a prior cesarean delivery were opting for a vaginal birth.

During that time, concern about possible complications, especially uterine rupture, had seemingly diminished to an almost blasé attitude. On the other hand, some doctors complained that they felt forced by third-party payers to push patients into accepting vaginal birth after cesarean when a patient didn't fully understand the risks. Some insurance companies developed consent forms for liability that were so intimidating that some women denied the procedure.

Referring again to the article in the *New England Journal of Medicine,* Sachs et al. point out that an elective repeat C-section costs approximately $900 more than a safe vaginal birth in a labor unit. But the issue of cost grows more complex if the birth has complications. If a woman attempts to give birth vaginally and fails, later needing a C-section, the cost is estimated at $3,000 more than a normal vaginal delivery. Should she experience a uterine rupture, she'll face another $4,000 in immediate medical costs, plus $2,000 more for her child. Even though that extra cost would devastate the uninsured patient, the odds of it occurring are low enough to make an increase in VBACs economically motivating for the large insurance company.

In 1998, the *Los Angeles Times* reported that Los Angeles County paid $24 million to settle forty-nine claims on behalf of mothers and children who had died or been injured at county hospitals as a result of complications of a trial of labor or vaginal delivery after a cesarean delivery.

Due to the inherent risks to patients and their unborn babies and in part due to legal risks, the pendulum is swinging back toward cesarean births as a valid choice after a previous cesarean. Nationwide VBAC rates have fallen 17 percent since 1996. ACOG and most other societies state that VBAC should only be undertaken if an immediate emergency cesarean, if necessary, could be accomplished within minutes. It has now been shown that the uterine scar rupture rate is higher than had been thought for many years, and is probably around the 1 percent range. A few further factors that might increase this rupture risk have been identified: (1) the time between babies (if less than two years between the two deliveries, the risk for rupture appears to be higher); and (2) a consideration of the way the uterus incision had been closed during the first cesarean.

Traditionally, the uterus had always been closed in two layers after a cesarean. About five years ago the trend changed, and it became common for the incision to be closed in only one layer. It made intuitive sense that it would not matter since it was believed that the main effect of suturing the uterus was to only stop the bleeding. We know that the sutures, even if pulled quite tight during the cesarean, become loose very quickly (within two days or so) as a result of the very quick shrinkage in size of the postpartum uterus. Anyway, as a result of this, it was believed that a one-layer closing that stopped bleeding was as good as the more traditional two-layer closing. This idea and habit spread quickly. Then more recent research found that there might be an increased rupture rate of one-layer closed scars in subsequent cesareans. So the trend is heading back to the two-layer closing.

Induction of labor is another high-risk area for scar rupture. If prostaglandins are used for cervical ripening, the risk of scar rupture is fifteen times higher than for a spontaneous labor. As a result, many gynecologists will not use prostaglandins but rather do a cesarean, if pregnancy termination is indicated. Unfortunately labor induction often requires prostaglandins if there is going to be any hope of success.

In my own practice, I've noticed that more and more women are choosing elective cesarean after previous cesarean. They feel the attempt at vaginal delivery is not worth the risk of uterine rupture with its potentially catastrophic results. The fact that certain obstetrical and government entities may encourage VBAC means little to them. When they hear there is a 1 percent risk of a scar dehiscence or rupture, with potentially serious morbidity or mortality to the baby, as well as the fact that only 60 to 65 percent of women will succeed at VBAC, I've found that most are simply not interested. Of course this is a generalization, as there are women who are adamant that they want a vaginal birth. I encourage them that their decision is the right one for *them*, provided they have all the information.

Medical Liability

Another driving force behind the increasing cesarean section rate is the litigation atmosphere that pervades our society, and the mistaken belief that a bad outcome necessarily implies that someone is to blame. The public has the impression (partly created by the medical establishment, and partly by the media), that medical science has overcome clinical disease and reproductive problems to a degree that we can, in reality, only wish for. These raised expectations create a situation where anything other than the perfect outcome is just unacceptable. It should be obvious what impact this has had on obstetric practice.

Government reports indicate that the number of malpractice claims filed against physicians nationwide rose at an average annual rate of 10 percent in the 1980s. Malpractice premiums rose over the same period by 113 percent for specialists in obstetrics and gynecology. In response, some obstetricians started practicing "defensive medicine," or the use of diagnostic tests and procedures that may not have been employed if not for the fear of litigation.

A New York state-focused study, supported in part by the Agency for Health Care Policy and Research (AHCPR), maintains that nearly one-fourth of all cesarean sections examined were the result of defensive medicine. Mothers with prior C-sections and cases of abnormal labor were excluded. The analysis revealed that nearly 7 percent of an overall C-section rate of 28 percent was due to fear of malpractice suits. Slightly more than 4 percent of this increase was a direct effect, and 2.2 percent was an indirect effect of increased EFM and increased diagnosis of fetal distress and resulting C-sections.

In January 2001, the *Los Angeles Times* reported that the number-one reason for lawsuits against obstetricians and gynecologists is a failure to perform a *timely* C-section. As a result, some physicians feel the best way to prevent a lawsuit is to go to a cesarean sooner than later.

Non Stress Test and Electronic Fetal Monitoring

I now want to discuss a development in modern obstetrics that has been of great importance, but which also has led to great problems in regard to the issue at hand, namely the decision to perform a cesarean section or not. This is the so-called non stress test (NST) prior to labor (before contractions exert "stress" on the placenta and fetus, including the fetus's oxygen supply), as well as EFM, which is the same test but is done in labor, with contractions.

The NST was introduced nearly thirty years ago without *any* scientific proof that it delivers on its claim: safer labors and more healthy newborns. There have literally been dozens if not hundreds of studies looking into the effects of NST on labor outcome. So far the only scientifically validated effect has been a lower rate of neonatal convulsions. Although this is certainly a serious problem if it occurs, the difference between those babies that were electronically monitored and those that were not was small, and the long-term outcomes were identical. There were no differences in cerebral palsy or other mental outcomes in any study that I am aware of to date. As a result of this, most obstetrical societies state that it is appropriate to monitor low-risk babies with nonelectronic, or noncontinuous, monitoring. In spite of this, it is almost impossible to get the monitors off of these low-risk patients. The monitor is here to stay. It is too easy, too apparently reassuring to the nurse and the prospective parents and family, and has an almost hypnotic quality to it.

Few understand that electronic fetal monitoring leads to increased cesarean section rates. Consider that abnormal heart rates are so common as to be almost normal. Although there are well-known classic abnormalities that might indicate a compromised fetus, the majority is spurious and of no real concern. Obstetricians are well aware that 40 percent of all test strips supposedly indicating fetal distress are incorrect. A cesarean section done for this indication most commonly leads to a baby that screams its state of non-jeopardized health to the world the moment it gets delivered through the cesarean incision.

Some heart rate abnormalities certainly have a more likely predictive value in diagnosing real fetal compromise. These are not always easy to separate from the spurious ones, and experience and training are required to differentiate. There are some helpful techniques that might help one to separate them. These include:

1. Fetal scalp blood sampling. This is a method of obtaining a little droplet of blood from the fetus's scalp and examining the oxygen content, as well as the pH of the fetus's blood. If it is normal, the fetus is almost certainly in excellent shape. For reasons to be explained, as well as the fact that it can be difficult, time consuming, and uncomfortable to the mother, many obstetricians do not bother with it and simply call for a cesarean section.

2. Fetal oxygenation assessment. This is a relatively new method of measuring the oxygenation of the fetus's blood with a special sensor through its skin. It is noninvasive, but is an expensive and seldom available technology that is still considered experimental.

But consider that the real-life situation is this: The obstetrician gets called to the labor room for fetal distress. Often this is the first contact with the patient and her family. As the OB walks in, the tension in the room is palpable. The family knows the fetal heart should be between the parameters the nurse has explained, and it is obvious to all that it is deviating from those parameters. Words like "fetal distress," "heart decelerations," or "slow heart rate" might have been spoken. They believe the fetus is at imminent risk, and the mere fact that the OB has been called in confirms their fears.

Now put yourself in the OB's shoes: The easiest way to reassure any human being is to tell that person that the situation is under control, and if not, that you know exactly what is going on, and that you will take immediate steps to regain control and solve the problem immediately. It is much more difficult to inform those present that there was no problem in the first place. One, you would be subtly humiliating the referring primary care physician and attending nurse; and two, everybody can see for themselves that the fetal heart is doing "funny" things, and they simply often don't believe you. Thus, not "solving the problem then and there" requires not only courage, but also determination, and unfortunately creates risk.

Nobody can predict the future. A fetus that might be perfectly fine one minute might indeed be at risk a while later. Should there be a "less than perfect" outcome in today's world where less than perfect is often just not acceptable, the OB will likely face those same parents in a court of law many years later, where lawyers scrutinize individual pieces of test tracing, and demand "yes" and "no" answers. It truly is a no-win situation.

So what often happens is this: Even though an OB knows that electronic fetal heart rate monitoring often leads to false warnings, and although it may be known that a particular warning is almost certainly false, it often is much, much easier to simply state that they will solve the problem immediately by delivering the baby by cesarean section within the next twenty minutes. In these cases, the parents are invariably overwhelmed with gratitude. Compare that with the situation of the OB stating (after possibly being called in for the second or third time to look at the strip, probably in the middle of the night) that everything is fine, the fetus is fine, and that the primary care physician or nurse, or both, are nervous for no reason. This, with an expectant father who is close to tears, a laboring woman who is consumed with worry, all because of a technology that promised the world, but delivered nothing at all.

Nobody ever accuses an OB of an unnecessary cesarean section when it is done for supposed fetal distress. But the reverse is all too common.

The point is this: Many cesarean sections are done for these nonmedical indications. As illustrated, these reasons are often the result of interpersonal situations and societal expectations and demands, that are putting the OB in an impossible position, where the way of least resistance is to be the hero, and "save" the baby from fetal distress.

In truth, there are some who use this situation for financial gain. There is nothing easier than to explain to new parents that an immediate cesarean section is required because a fetal strip shows some (though often false) deceleration of the fetal heart. There are *very* few people indeed that will not go along with this. Although this sounds unbelievable, one has to appreciate that electronically monitored fetal traces show a spectrum of characteristics, and the individual tolerance of OBs will differ. Training and experiences gained (or suffered) also will impact on the rapidity of a possible cesarean section. *However, the percentage of those who will do cesarean sections for purely financial reasons, is, I believe, small, but certainly not zero.*

Bucking the System

Indeed, cesarean section has become an easy way out in many situations. The danger exists that caregivers may resort to cesarean section in cases of minimally abnormal labor when, in fact, vaginal birth could be successfully accomplished. Some of the reasons for this might be to hide a lack of knowledge, to satisfy minor logistical problems or inconveniences, or to ensure daytime deliveries.

Physicians who are involved in labors while also trying to run an office at the same time may be significantly stressed when schedules are interrupted. I can well remember practicing in a small town and being called away from an office full of patients, some of whom have driven hours to see me. It is certainly difficult to wait out a prolonged second stage in this situation and not be influenced in your decision to use a forceps or vacuum for the delivery, due to factors other than the obstetrical situation alone. In smaller communities, the number of deliveries and their associated remuneration sometimes leave you with little alternative than to practice in this way. In larger communities, where the numbers of deliveries are sufficient, physicians can concentrate on obstetrical care on an on-call rotation. In this situation, the stress is significantly reduced, and the temptation for intervention lessened.

Whereas midwives spend the entire labor with their patients, physicians do not. This is the result of the medical system that was developed, rather than chosen. Physicians just cannot spend a lot of time with any single patient, and tend to be present only a few times during labor, or often only right at the end for the actual delivery. With the time restraints, the need to *do something* became paramount in their minds. Many of the ideas of putting time limits on certain parts of labor originally had little to do with science, and more to do with of this need to be active, and to be seen as being active. This certainly led to the development of some unnecessary interventions, the shunting aside of the traditional midwife's role, and serious conflict. Certainly, echoes of this can still be found today.

To a large degree, physicians are trapped in an inflexible system of maternity care where it is impossible to spend time. This "system" consists not only of the policies and practices in place in hospitals and institutions, but also in fee schedules, liability insurance rates, and remuneration systems that have developed in such a way that physicians have to see an inordinate number of patients to make their practices economically viable.

Take for example the current fee system in place in Canada. Midwives are paid a set rate for maternity care, or are allowed to bill privately at a level far exceeding the remuneration of their physician (even specialist physician) colleagues. Of course, the argument is made that physicians see more patients and therefore earn more. This is of course a circular argument. The fact remains that minimizing time spent per patient, as encouraged by this system, could potentially lead to unnecessary interventions. So in some sense, the accusation that physicians do unnecessary interventions is a legitimate concern.

Unfortunately, the situation becomes quite complicated as it pertains to the practice of consulting and primary care obstetrics. When I am on call as a specialist, I am asked to come in to assess a situation and give my verdict about whether we should continue as is, or whether something such as an instrumental intervention or cesarean should be done. The expectation that the specialist is going to *do something* that will relieve the fear and anxiety of the new parents to be is almost overwhelming. Stating that all should continue as before and that everything is in order is often met with paradoxical hostility. As the person knowing that "the buck stops here," this is not a comfortable situation to be in. As we have outlined previously, one can easily predict that if something were to go wrong in later stages of labor and delivery, that litigation might not be far off. Such is the lot of the obstetrician. Some (thankfully, the minority) obstetricians have responded to this no-win situation by simply throwing in the towel and stating that a cesarean is necessary. Similarly, instrumental vaginal deliveries might be chosen.

Although I honestly believe that most of today's physicians practice ethical medicine in light of current knowledge, and with the patients' best interests at heart, the system has developed in a way that makes some of the above problems inevitable.

Avoiding Unnecessary Cesarean Deliveries

I completely agree that we should be reducing unnecessary cesarean sections. By "unnecessary," I mean doing a cesarean for women who really want to have a vaginal delivery. This includes *every* woman who has entered the labor ward with the idea of delivering vaginally (with the exception of those who must have a cesarean for medical reasons). The labor room is *not* the place to discuss the effects of vaginal delivery on pelvic floor health. This should have been done *long* before that. I believe that there is ample opportunity to reduce the number of unnecessary cesarean sections through a few relatively simple changes.

1. Incorporate a discussion of the limitations of EFM in prenatal classes.
2. Make sure obstetrical caregivers can interpret electronic fetal monitor traces, and are keeping up to date with new thinking and developments in this regard. This is not only necessary for physicians, but also equally important for the obstetrical nurses. Better yet, stop monitoring low-risk laboring women with continuous electronic monitoring. The emphasis is on *low-risk*. I'm not suggesting continuous electronic monitoring doesn't have a place. But the use of it in *all* laboring women is an abuse of a technology that has caused thousands of women to be robbed of a desired vaginal delivery. I'm afraid, however, that it might be too late for this. EFM is currently so entrenched that the only way its use will probably diminish is if it gets replaced by a newer and better technology such as fetal blood oxygenation monitoring, computerized fetal heart rate interpretation, and others.
3. Make sure everyone involved in obstetrical care understands in *no* uncertain terms the limitations of electronic fetal monitoring, and the fact that a few variable decelerations, a temporary change in baseline, and many other commonly found so-called "abnormalities" do *not* mean that a cesarean is ultimately necessary. Set departmental guidelines requiring fetal scalp pH monitoring before resorting to cesarean for a diagnosis of fetal distress, if possible (it is not always possible—or reasonable—to do so).
4. Strongly discourage the use of cesarean section as a "cop-out" in situations like I have mentioned earlier in this chapter. This discouragement could be in the form of departmental peer reviews or strict guidelines. It is the norm that obstetrical practices vary tremendously, and so do the cesarean rates of different physicians. Nobody likes being "audited," however, and resistance to this idea can be expected.
5. Move to call groups or shared on-call systems, if possible. Here I mean that obstetricians do not necessarily deliver their own maternity patients when they come in, but that a group of obstetricians come together in a call group, and take turns to do call. The person who is on-call at that time delivers everybody's patients, and does not schedule any other work

> for that period of time. He/she is thus completely available, and has no incentive or pressure to "get it over with" so he/she can return to his/her other duties, etc. I know that this idea will come as a shock to many women. The very thought of *not* being delivered by your "own" doctor might even be unacceptable to many, at first reaction. Let's be honest: During most deliveries, the physician comes in at the last minute (having come in maybe once or twice during the course of labor), helps to deliver the baby and placenta, sutures, checks that everything is normal, and then leaves. It is the nurse that spends the majority of the time with the patient, and who really has the most intimate association with her. I'm *not* implying that I don't enjoy delivering my own patients. By nature, I'm quite an emotional person, and I've shed many tears of happiness with my patients after the baby has arrived safely. That feeling makes the practice of obstetrics so enjoyable. However, I've also made many new friends and acquaintances with people I met for the first time in the labor room.

I'll explain why I think this kind of obstetric practice leads to better medical care, and then I will let the reader make up her own mind.

I have worked in both setups. I practiced in small rural towns for almost seven years. I know the frustration of being on-call every second day and night (not to mention every second weekend!). I know what it means to have an office full of patients, some of whom have driven hours and have waited for a long time to see me, to be told I have to run out to deliver a baby, and might not be back. I know the stress this can put on a practitioner and the temptation to put the vacuum or the forceps on to "get it over with." I know how one can sometimes convince oneself that there really *is* an indication for an emergency cesarean section. I know the stress on family life when that social function you and your partner have waited for so long invariably gets disrupted by the inconsiderate baby, or when you have a patient that just *might* go into labor on the very evening of a once-a-year function. Again, the wish to get the job done so you can leave can become a danger not only to the ethical management of your patient, but also to the practitioner's mental health.

Then there's the issue of sleep deprivation, and the associated decrease in effective functioning. Many people seem oblivious to the fact that physicians get tired, sleep deprived, irritable, depressed, etc., when they are overworked. I do believe this abuse problem is bigger in socialized medical systems like that of Canada, and probably the NHS, than in private systems in the United States. The interesting thing is that most professions have strict standards of maximum work hours after which time off is obligatory. Pilots have to hand over, truck drivers have to pull over, police and other rescue workers have to go home (I'm not talking about crisis situations). By contrast, physicians can (and do) work for twenty-four to thirty-six hours without stopping. One-hundred-hour weeks are not uncommon. As a patient, you demand and expect the best care possible. You expect your physician to take care of you, and to make decisions that are in your best interests. You might have no idea that your doctor is running on empty. Maybe he/she has had two hours sleep in the last forty-eight hours. Any reasonable person will see that this situation can easily lead to bad obstetrical care—and ultimately a rising cesarean section rate and the *then* justified accusation from midwives that obstetricians are doing too many unnecessary interventions.

Compare the aforementioned situation with the call-group system. Each physician works for a defined period of time. Each doctor knows exactly when he/she will come off duty. During this time the doctor accepts that he/she will be busy and will have no other arrangement that could conflict. There is absolutely no need to rush anything. You have to be there, and whether the baby comes now, or an hour or two later it makes no difference. There is no need or temptation for "early" intervention or cesarean.

Since I've worked in both systems, I can honestly say I truly believe the call-group system of shared care leads to better quality care for my patients.

Unfortunately, it can work only if there is a critical mass of obstetricians to share the call, and it is thus only possible in larger centers and cities. It is also necessary that the call group exert some measure of monitoring over its members' practices, so that each member can honestly reassure their patients that they will get the same level of care that their own physician could have given, except for the fact that the personal connection isn't there. In Calgary (a city with almost a million people) where I live and practice, this shared call-group type of obstetrical care, with in-house call (OB stays in the hospital and is immediately available for the full period of time he/she is on call) has become the standard of care in all Calgary Regional Health Authority hospitals.

Safety of Today's Cesarean

It is well recognized that cesarean section in general carries more risk than a normal vaginal birth. The problem comes in recognizing what is a "normal" vaginal birth, and which cesarean deliveries should be compared to vaginal deliveries.

Usually (almost all studies that have looked at this), all vaginal deliveries and *all* cesareans are simply lumped together. I will argue that this is patently ridiculous. By far the majority of vaginal deliveries are for healthy young women with normal pregnancies. In today's medical-legal climate, as well as with improvements in perinatal care, it has almost become the norm that many complicated obstetrical cases, or cases with significant maternal compromise are delivered by cesarean. This by itself makes a powerful argument for the safety of the cesarean operation. However, it should be clear that the studies are thus not comparing apples to apples. The number of cesareans done for healthy, well-hydrated women who are fasting and don't have some serious or potentially serious medical or surgical disorder is very small, compared to cesareans done for women with certain medical problems, for instance those who are in labor for a very long time or those situations where serious imminent disaster forces an immediate intervention. Many of these women are dehydrated, demoralized, exhausted, overworked, and have a stomach that is full of food and thus would universally be considered to be of higher risk.

In spite of these facts, the cesarean operation is a remarkably safe one. The available studies seem to indicate that the risks to the mother are about between two to four times that of vaginal delivery. Keep in mind what I said about comparing apples to oranges. There are some indications that the situation with the completely elective (scheduled) cesarean done for the otherwise healthy mother is different.

One large multicenter worldwide study recently found basically no difference between the outcomes for mothers who delivered breech babies vaginally versus those that delivered by planned cesarean section. This same study also found without doubt that term, singleton, breech babies are better off delivered by cesarean than by the vaginal route. This has been suspected for a long time, and the situation on the ground was that of a slow change to universal cesarean deliveries of breech babies anyway. Since this study was prematurely stopped as a result of the dramatic differences found, it would be a brave obstetrician indeed who would recommend vaginal delivery of a term breech baby. The study did not look at situations of premature breech babies, or at the situation where the second of twins is breech. This last situation especially, might be different.[2]

Anyway, in this study, most (not all, since some women enter labor before the date of the scheduled C-section and end up being an emergency C-section) women had a planned, elective cesarean section. The study was designed to look at the perinatal (fetus and newborn) and neonatal (after delivery) outcome. The finding that the mothers' outcomes were the *same* was a surprise.

In my opinion, this is one of the few prospective studies where apples were compared with apples. And guess what—the apples were found to be the same!

Some studies have "proven" that cesarean delivery is more dangerous for the mother than vaginal delivery, and that as such it is imperative to reduce cesarean section rates. The maternal morbidity (complication rate) was found in some of these to be up to four times that of vaginal delivery. If one looks at the studies however, it becomes clear that in almost all cases, all cesareans were thrown together, and there was seldom an attempt to select purely elective cesareans in healthy women. A few of the studies looking at elective cesareans specifically found the overall differences in maternal mortality and morbidity to be very comparable to vaginal delivery.

My problem is *not* with the findings of those studies that found a higher risk. Actually, I can completely accept their findings and conclusions and still make the case that cesarean is in fact a very safe operation. I totally accept that an emergency cesarean section for complicated medical, obstetrical, and surgical problems and complications would yield a group of mothers (and babies) who had more complications and "bad" outcomes on average than a much larger group of (mostly) healthy women with normal pregnancies and healthy fetuses, where cesarean was not deemed necessary. This seems so obvious that having to state the fact seems ludicrous. However, the blanket statements and interpretations that usually follow findings like these are disturbing. Some people seem unable to separate these cesareans in their minds from the elective cesareans as I have described them.

Having stated all of this, it is still likely that even completely elective (as defined) cesarean sections might carry a higher risk to the mother than vaginal delivery. Cesarean section is, after all, a relatively major surgery, and the abdominal cavity is entered, which always causes some risk.

In an editorial entitled, "What Is the Correct Cesarean Rate and How Do We Get There?" authors Edward G. Peskin, M.D., and Gabrielle M. Reine, M.D., say:

> One clear difficulty with a single cesarean delivery rate for all is that physicians vary with respect to their patient populations and, in turn, with their patients' risk factors for requiring a cesarean delivery. Obviously, obstetricians caring for women with multiple gestations, chronic medical conditions, and preterm labor cannot be expected to uphold the same rate as providers with practices composed primarily of women with full-term, uncomplicated pregnancies. This rate is, therefore, a constantly changing, moving target. A rate of 22% would have been incorrect in 1900 when a cesarean delivery involved significant maternal morbidity and mortality. Because of more effective antibiotics, carefully screened blood transfusions, and improvements in anesthesia and surgical techniques, the risks involved with a cesarean delivery have been markedly decreased. The safety of the surgery has allowed for examination of the potential benefits to both mother and baby. Some are obvious, such as when a delivery is performed for a placenta previa or a fetus with acidosis. Other long-term benefits may not be as readily apparent, such as the prevention of incontinence and pelvic organ prolapse. As our knowledge and technology advance, the cesarean delivery will likely become an even safer procedure, the accuracy of intrapartum fetal assessment will improve and we will hopefully be able to better select candidates for a trial of labor.[3]

Additionally, I need to stress that any risks of cesarean delivery should be put into the perspective of the short-term versus the long-term risks, as well as the potential of having an impact on future reproduction. For this reason I would argue that the risks on reproduction should be seen in terms of the woman's future reproductive wishes. There is a complete difference between an older woman wanting only one or two children (increasingly the norm), and younger women or those who want more than two children. This has never been addressed in any study.

THE DEMOGRAPHIC QUOTIENT

Women are having fewer and fewer children and having them later in life. For example, the current mean for Canadian mothers is nearly 1.6 children. Another trend is having the first baby later in life. Couples frequently know exactly how many children they plan to have and undergo permanent contraceptive methods when they reach their target. A recent article in the *Los Angeles Times* reports that hospital officials attribute the rising cesarean section rates, in part, to more births to first-time mothers in their thirties and forties who are more likely to encounter complications that lead to cesarean sections. These older, first-time mothers often gain more weight during pregnancy and have bigger babies, factors that can increase the difficulty of vaginal birth.

American Medical News quotes one expert as saying, "What we're doing is trying to lower the cesarean delivery rate at a time when vaginal birth is becoming harder for many women. The result will be more prolonged labor, more complications and more dissatisfied patients."[4]

As a result of women choosing to have fewer children, the negative effects of cesarean section for repetitive pregnancies and future births is significantly reduced. However, this is one of the main reasons cited for the need to reduce cesarean section rates. Obviously, there is a major difference between women who plan their pregnancies and know how many children they want, and those who know that they want many children. For this latter group, the higher risk of subsequent and multiple operations, and the inherent risks of the scarred uterus for future pregnancies, will obviously outweigh many of the benefits of elective cesarean birth. But as shown, this group is becoming a minority and is likely to remain so for the foreseeable future.

Women today can expect to live a major portion of their lives after they have finished their childbearing. Life expectancy in the Western world is the highest it has ever been in human history and is still climbing. Consequently, and due to a decreasing birthrate, the time that women in the Western world spend pregnant, as a percentage of their lifespan, is the lowest it has ever been. Any negative effect of childbirth on a woman's future, in quality-of-life terms, is thus more important today than it has ever been in history.

Women live more active lives with increasing participation in sports, business, and all walks of life into old age. Therefore, long-term complications of vaginal birth, such as urinary and fecal incontinence, can be disastrous to productivity and the overall quality of life. These disorders can no longer be viewed as the maladies of "little old ladies." There was a time that women were almost expected to suffer these symptoms in embarrassed silence. Today, they rightfully do not and cannot put up with it anymore. Unfortunately for them, it often means major, sometimes repetitive and expensive surgery with no guarantees of success.

Due to demographic and lifestyle changes, as well as future increasing knowledge about the pelvic floor and the effects of vaginal childbirth on its components, I believe that the drive to reduce cesarean section rates will fail in the long term. The protection of the pelvic floor is destined to become a major indication for elective cesarean births in the very near future.

NOTES

1. B. P. Sachs, C. Kobelin, M. A. Castro, et al., "The Risks of Lowering the Cesarean-Delivery Rate," *New England Journal of Medicine* 340 (1999): 54–57.

2. M. E. Hannah, "Planned Cesarean Section versus Planned Vaginal Birth for Breech Presentation at Term: A Randomized Multicentre Trial," *Lancet* 356, no. 9239 (October 2000): 1375–83.

3. Edward G. Peskun and Gabrielle M. Reine, "What Is the Correct Cesarean Role and How Do We Get There?" *Obstetric Gynecology Survey* 57, no. 4 (April 2002): 189–90.

4. *American Medical News* 44, no. 20 (May 28, 2001): 25.

EIGHTEEN
Cesarean Birth
The Facts

I believe that protection of the pelvic floor is an acceptable indication for an elective cesarean. This statement would imply that a fully informed patient has weighed all the facts, including the possible risks and complications, before she makes a decision. But it is also my opinion that the moment a patient enters labor with the intention of having a vaginal delivery, protection of the pelvic floor, as an indication for cesarean, falls away completely and permanently. To resort to this indication at a later stage during labor would, in my view, be an inappropriate attempt to justify doing a cesarean section for the sake of convenience (in the absence of another solid indication). These issues are not something that should be discussed during labor, but rather during pregnancy, when there is enough time to weigh all the consequences rationally.

TECHNIQUE OF CESAREAN SECTION

I was recently asked a question by a patient that made me realize once more how many misconceptions abound relating to various medical interventions. The patient asked me how long her "cut" abdominal muscles would take to heal. As I was already busy working on this manuscript, the question was quite an eye-opener. I immediately decided that a short section explaining the technique of a cesarean section was imperative.

The answer to the above question is that *no* abdominal muscles are in fact cut. The only muscle that is cut is the uterus.

The steps in a cesarean are basically (with some minor variation) as follows:

The skin of the lower abdominal wall is incised in a transverse direction just above the pubic hairline, in the majority of cases (side to side rather than up and down). A longitudinal (up and down) incision is seldom employed. Just under the skin, a layer of fat is found which is easily separated to reach the next layer. The reader will recognize this next type of layer since it is a dense shiny white layer of fascia called the rectus fascia. Like the pelvic fascia, this is a connective tissue layer that surrounds the rectus abdominal muscles and offers support, attachment, and strength. This fascia layer is incised to expose the two rectus abdominal muscles which are big muscles running from the rib cage to the pubic bone. These are the main muscles employed to do sit-ups. The two muscles meet in the midline where they are sometimes fused but quite often, however, they are separated as the result of the stretching from the distended uterus. These muscles are now separated (no abdominal muscles are actually cut during cesarean section. The two rectus muscles are just spread apart. This is one of the most common misconceptions) and pulled to the sides to create a space between them.

After this space has been created, the only layers covering the uterus are thin fascia and the peritoneum. The peritoneal layer is a very thin membranelike layer, which can be described as the lining of the abdominal cavity. After this layer is penetrated, the uterus will lie directly in view. A second layer of peritoneum, which is also incised and pushed out of the way, usually covers the lower segment of the uterus where the incision will be made. This simple part of a cesarean section helps to prevent injuries to the bladder, which lies on top of the lowest part of the uterus and the immediate vagina. Some people argue that this step increases the risk of future adhesions of the bladder onto the lower part of the uterus, which might cause problems during a future operation like another cesarean or perhaps a future hysterectomy. As a result, there are increasing numbers of obstetricians who leave this step out.

After the bladder has been pushed to safety, the next step is to incise the uterus. The incision in the uterine wall is also made transversely, and it is made in the lower segment of the uterus, just above the cervix, which is the thinnest part. The incision is usually started with a scalpel but usually completed by manual stretching. This is done to prevent injury to the immediately underlying infant. The baby is then delivered by guiding its head into the opening with one hand while the assistant exerts pressure on the uterine fundus (top of the uterus).

After delivery, the baby is handed to the pediatrician, after which the placenta is removed by manually grasping it and pulling it through the incision. At this point the antibiotic, as well as a drug (oxytocin) to ensure contraction of the uterus, is usually administrated by the anesthetist. Suturing of the uterine incision commences immediately and can be done in one or more layers. The peritoneal layers can be sutured or left open. I personally am of the school that believes that there is no benefit in suturing the peritoneum in most cases and that it does not make a big difference one way or the other. The final two layers that need closing are the rectus sheath, and of course the skin. The rectus sheath is the most important layer (not surprisingly—it's fascia!) and needs to be sutured with strong material. The skin can be closed with sutures, staples, or various other methods, none of which have significant advantages over the other. It is sometimes necessary, especially in subsequent cesarean births, to place a suction drain underneath the rectus sheath. This is to prevent the collection of serum or blood in this area, which could then become a site for infection. These drains would typically stay in for twelve to twenty-four hours. The urinary catheter and IV are usually also removed at the same time.

The scar after cesarean birth is usually not unsightly and in fact is often difficult to see. This depends to a large degree on the patient's skin type, the presence or absence of infection in the wound, and of course the location and length of the incision. The underlying skin will lose some of its pliability, which sometimes causes an overlying fat roll, if present, to curl around the scar. Although some women complain of this, it needs to be pointed out that most women who have had children have some signs of stretching of the abdominal wall, for instance stretch marks or some extra skin laxity. Be proud of it!

It is certainly true that a cesarean birth is more impersonal and certainly more "medical" than a natural vaginal birth. This cannot be changed. With newer spinal anesthetic techniques, however, the mother-to-be can now participate in the event to the degree that she will be able to hear exactly what is going on, including baby's first cry. The husband or significant other can also be part of the happy event and can even watch the delivery itself. The baby is usually handed to the father almost immediately, who takes the baby over to the mother for the first cuddle.

Risks of Cesarean Birth

As we have said, there are risks involved with any surgical procedure. This section will cover the risks involved with cesarean birth, and importantly, *contrast the difference in risk potential between emergency cesarean birth and elective cesarean birth.*

Many articles compare the safety of cesarean birth to that of vaginal delivery. Most of these articles are somewhat dated, but they had found cesarean section to be the more hazardous option. Consensus opinion estimated the mortality risk to be two to five times higher for cesarean section than for vaginal delivery. Most of this data is from the 1960s and 1970s, however, and is thus questionable.

There are also studies that question the perception that cesarean mortality is higher than that of vaginal delivery. One study by Sachs et al. found that cesarean-related mortality was lower than that of vaginal delivery. This was in spite of the fact that the study made no distinction between emergency and elective cesarean sections. The cesarean related mortality was 5.8 per 100,000 births.[1] The authors concluded that the mortality risk was similar between vaginally delivered and cesarean delivered women, all else being equal. It is well known that emergency cesarean is more risky than elective cesarean, and this risk differential has been calculated to be at least 1.7 (nonelective cesarean section is at least 1.7 times more risky than elective cesarean section).

One other large study, the recently completed "Term Breech Trial," has also made the unexpected observation that there was no difference in outcomes between the cesarean section and the vaginally delivered women. I quote directly: "Caesarean sections had no impact on maternal health, but are beneficial for the well-being of breech babies. Under a planned caesarean policy, for every additional 14 caesarean sections undertaken, one baby is saved from death or serious morbidity."[2]

But the fact remains that as elective cesarean section becomes safer, almost (or already) reaching that of vaginal deliveries for healthy women, the risks of failed vaginal delivery with resultant emergency cesarean will increase the overall risk to women.

However, let's look at some of the recognized risks of cesarean section. Some of these will be influenced by patient-specific factors like age, concurrent medical conditions, number of previous cesareans, and other abdominal surgery.

As a general rule, the safest cesarean will be that in young, healthy, nonobese women who have not had previous abdominal surgery, and who can be mobilized (gotten out of bed) quickly.

The most common severe complications leading to maternal death after cesarean section are anesthetic complications, infections with sepsis, thromboembolic (blood clot) problems especially pulmonary embolism (blood clot in lung), and bleeding. It is extremely important to note that the studies, which compared the risks of cesarean sections, lumped all cesareans together. There are almost no studies that looked only at *elective* cesareans in healthy patients. Since most cesarean sections are done for abnormal pregnancies or labors, including some severe medical conditions, there will almost certainly be major differences in risk between the emergency cesarean and the elective one. We'll examine some of these risks in more detail.

Anesthetic Complications

One of the major problems with emergency cesarean section is the fact that patients do not have empty stomachs. They have either eaten, drank fluids, or both, relatively shortly before the surgery becomes necessary. A full stomach is one of the most serious risk factors for general anesthetics, and in most nonemergency situations anesthetists would postpone the surgery. The problem is that there is an increased risk of inhalation (breathing in) of stomach content, which is an extremely dangerous situation. With an elective cesarean birth, the patients are fasting.

Further developments over the last decade include greater experience with epidural and spinal anesthesia. Spinal anesthesia is a reliable and easily learned anesthetic technique. It works quickly, provides a dense block, and involves only a single quick injection into the cerebrospinal fluid (fluid column surrounding the spinal nerves). In my opinion, it is by far the preferred method.

Unfortunately, the more common epidural anesthesia has multiple disadvantages compared to spinal anesthesia. First of all, it takes a long time to work. Or, it might not work at all, or may not provide a block which is dense enough, and so a higher dose of local anesthetic is used with more associated risks of toxicity. The needle used in epidural is thicker that with spinal, and if the needle accidentally punctures the dura mater layer of the spinal canal, the patient has a much higher chance of having a significant "postspinal headache."

With both these methods the patient stays awake, although if preferred she can be heavily sedated. A spouse or significant other is commonly allowed to sit with her, to share in the experience and provide support.

In comparison to a general anesthetic, spinal anesthesia is definitely preferable and, as a rule, general anesthesia should be used only as an exception.

Potential Side Effects and Complications of Spinal Anesthesia

1. ***Postdural puncture headache (spinal headache).*** This distressing problem is a result of a slow leakage of spinal fluid from the puncture site. In its mild form, it is a nuisance only; but in its more severe presentations it can be disabling, and the sufferer is forced to stay flat on her back. Lying down relieves this headache almost immediately, for reasons that are well known but fall outside of the scope of our discussion. The risk of this problem is approximately 1 percent. One has to keep in mind that the same risk exists for epidurals. Although the absolute risk in epidurals is somewhat lower, since the needle in an epidural should not penetrate completely into the

spinal fluid column. If it does occur, chances are that the degree of headache will be worse. The reason for this is the thicker needle used for epidural establishment. One should consider the fact that up to 70 or 80 percent of women in labor, with expectations of vaginal birth, receive epidural anesthetics.

2. ***Nerve damage.*** This major complication is fortunately extremely rare, and also occurs with epidurals. A study published in 1995 by Scott and Tunstall reported forty-six cases of neurological complications after 122,989 spinal and epidural anesthetics.[3] There were no reports of permanent disability, however, and complete recovery occurred in all cases.

3. ***High block.*** This rare but serious complication involves a rising level of nerve blockage, which could eventually cause loss of consciousness and is potentially life threatening. As long as the problem is recognized in good time the anesthetic could be converted to a full general anesthetic and the necessary resuscitation measures instituted. The important thing here, obviously, is to have an adequately trained anesthetist.

4. ***Backache.*** There seems to be no evidence of a relationship between spinal anesthesia and long-term backache.

5. ***Infection and hematoma.*** Although potentially serious, this is fortunately rare. A serious infection after a spinal anesthetic could lead to meningitis. Hematoma (blood clot) formation could cause pressure on the spinal canal. This extremely rare complication has been found in approximately one in 505,000 epidurals. The risk is even lower in spinals, as a result of the thinner needle used.

6. ***Shivering and itching.*** Again, these symptoms occur in both spinals and epidurals, but are less likely to occur in spinal anesthesia. The exact cause is unknown, but it occurs in about 10 percent of *normal* labors. The itching is a result of histamine release due to opioids (medications similar to morphine), which are added to the blocking agent to provide postoperative pain relief and to reduce the dose of blocking agent needed for adequate anesthesia. Interestingly, many women complain of itching of their nose tips.

7. ***Drop in blood pressure.*** This common occurrence can be prevented, or rapidly treated, if diagnosed early. It results from the opening up of large numbers of small blood vessels in the areas of the body (lower body) that are blocked. These blood vessels normally have an inherent tone (continuous state of contraction keeping their diameters small), which is lost as a result of the blockage of their own small nerves. With the sudden opening up of millions of small vessels, the average pressure in the vascular system drops. It is for this reason that most anesthetists will "top up" the fluid volume in a patient's vascular system by giving intravenous fluids before doing the spinal or epidural. Again, having an anesthetist with adequate experience and training cannot be stressed enough.

INFECTION

Infection is a possible complication of any operation. When we are dealing with elective surgery, however, this becomes an important factor to consider. One of the reasons for maternal deaths in the various studies was severe infection. These could be wound infections, intrauterine infections, pneumonia, or various other infections. As already mentioned, keep in mind that these studies lumped together all cesarean sections, regardless of the indication. A large percentage of these had risk factors for infection that makes the data invalid if looking at elective cesareans only. One of the well-known high risk factors for infection after vaginal or cesarean birth is having ruptured membranes for a long time ("ruptured membranes" means the water has broken, something that often occurs early in labor, either spontaneously, or induced). This creates an open passage from the vulva and vagina to the uterus. Every instrumentation and vaginal examination increases the risk of infection as a result of bacteria being pushed into the uterine cavity. Cesareans done after prolonged labor thus differ in a substantial way from the electively performed procedure with intact membranes.

Most women who consider an elective cesarean section for protection of their pelvic floor would not be likely to have serious medical or obstetrical complications, as these would become the overriding factors to direct the care and decisions made. Although there is little data to prove the point, it is logical to assume that these healthy patients would have a substantially lower risk of infection. Since spinal anesthesia is the preferred method, the risk of pneumonia can be substantially reduced as well. Pneumonia is a significant risk of general anesthetics, as a result of the potential inhalation of stomach content, as well as the mechanical ventilation (mechanical breathing) employed during the general anesthetic.

It has been adequately proven that a dose of antibiotics reduces the risk of infection after cesarean. Although not routinely given to all cesareans by every obstetrician, it has been shown to make a significant difference even in elective cases. I would recommend a single dose of intravenous antibiotics during the operation immediately after the baby is delivered. Giving it at that point prevents the baby from being exposed. Concern might arise about this apparent increase in antibiotic use. In my opinion, this is a nonissue. Current recommendations in North America, which are practiced throughout the world, show that approximately 40 percent of normally laboring women receive intravenous antibiotics during labor. The reason for the application of antibiotics is to prevent a serious infection caused by a certain organism called group B streptococcus. This organism has the potential to cause severe maternal infection, and moreover, to severely affect the newborn baby. It is recommended that all screen-positive women or all women with risk factors for this problem should receive antibiotics in labor. Since approximately 40 percent of women are colonized with this organism in their vaginas, they should thus be given antibiotics. These antibiotics are given throughout labor and multiple doses are usually employed to which the babies are obviously exposed. Other pregnant women who routinely receive antibiotics are those who go into premature labor. It is obvious that the use of antibiotics in pregnancy and labor is very common, and the application of a single prophylactic preoperative dose before elective cesarean birth might in reality decrease the total antibiotic dosage exposure, given a large enough cesarean birth rate.

Concern has been expressed in the last number of years about the potential increase of organisms that are resistant to multiple antibiotics. This is certainly of great concern to obstetricians and all physicians. Fortunately, this has not yet become a widespread problem. As argued above, higher numbers of elective cesareans will make no substantial difference to the induction of antibiotic resistance and may even have a paradoxical protective effect. Since the numbers will be relatively small in relation to the overall birth rate, however, I anticipate that there will be no real impact.

Infection with resistant organisms after cesarean birth is of more concern. The same could be said for *any* surgery, especially surgery that has no immediate life-threatening indications. Indeed, if this argument is used to restrict elective cesarean births, other commonly performed elective surgeries, such as cosmetic surgery, would be equally unjustifiable. For the time being, at any rate, this need not be a major concern in the decision-making process. Physicians should be aware of the incidence of these organisms in their specific hospitals and this is something that needs to be discussed between the patient and her physician. Recent and foreseen breakthroughs in ways to overcome the penicillin resistance of some bacteria might again make this less of a concern.

Thromboembolic Problems

The fragility of our connective tissues, especially in relation to blood vessels and to our thin-walled veins, is a constant reminder to me of our mortality and the thin line between life and death. The integrity of our blood vessels prevents us from bleeding to death, and equally important is the intactness of our blood-clotting mechanisms. Without this finely balanced and fascinating system, we would either instantaneously bleed from every pore, or our blood would immediately coalesce into a firm and gel-like clot. Neither of these scenarios is compatible with life.

The clotting mechanism, simplistically, consists of the functions of platelets, the clotting factors, fibrinogen, and various anticlotting agents. It is obvious that these proclotting and anticlotting factors must keep a delicate balance, to prevent inappropriate clotting, but at the same time must protect us from exsanguinating (bleeding to death) in the event of tissue injury. This balance can be influenced by many different causes, the best known is smoking (smoking has a proclotting effect). Various diseases and genetically determined disorders can also influence this system.

The pregnant woman is at a substantially increased risk of thromboembolic events as a result of the physiological changes in the blood clotting mechanisms that are associated with pregnancy. The risk of bloodclots in pregnancy is about six times that of the nonpregnant state. In fact, thromboembolism is the most common cause of maternal mortality. A cesarean definitely increases the risk, just like any surgery. Blood clots in the legs, called deep vein thrombosis and even clots in the lungs, called pulmonary embolisms, are serious events that occur more frequently in the pregnant than in the nonpregnant population. This increased risk is mostly due to a significant increase in many of the proclotting factors and fibrinogen in pregnancy. There are also certain well-known medical conditions that increase this risk even further. Unfortunately, these conditions are often not known to be present until unmasked by an acute thrombotic event. Major surgery, such as a cesarean, increases the risk.

Immobilization is known to be a major causal factor involved in thrombosis, especially after surgery. It is less of a factor for healthy women who opt for elective cesarean births than for those women who undergo an emergency cesarean section after a prolonged labor during which they were confined to bed. These emergency cases are often dehydrated, as a result of insufficient intake and of the increased fluid loss during rapid breathing and intensive muscle action that usually accompanies labor. In the elective case, the patient is usually healthy, was mobile immediately prior to the procedure, and although having fasted for a predetermined period of time, is usually not dehydrated. Any anesthetist worth his salt will replenish the patient's intravascular volume to ensure she is not dehydrated. Since the elective cesarean patients are usually less tired than those who underwent emergency surgery, in addition to being well motivated and fully informed patients, it is usually easier to motivate the elective cases to mobilize (get out of bed) after cesarean. It is always a pity if a patient had a failed forceps delivery and subsequent emergency cesarean, since on top of everything else, she often will have soreness from an episiotomy and the cesarean incision.

Since immobilization and dehydration are two of the most serious risk factors for thrombosis, I believe that the risk for healthy women having an elective cesarean birth is significantly lower than the level published in most articles. As mentioned before, these articles do not take into consideration the differences between the elective cases and the emergency ones. I suspect these differences to be so great as to almost make comparisons and extrapolations invalid.

Preventing thromboembolic complications of surgery has become an important aspect of preoperative as well as postoperative care of all surgical patients. In gynecological, general, and orthopedic surgery, the risk is especially high and steps are taken according to certain protocols and indications to lower that risk. In cases where patients are deemed to be at higher risk, methods employed might include stockings, leg bandaging, automatic compression stockings, or heparin, which is a drug used to prevent and treat blood clots. The drug is most often given as subcutaneous injections (superficial skin injections) prior to or immediately after surgery, and usually for as long as the patient is immobilized. It is well known that this drug does not cross the placenta and thus would not affect the fetus in any way. The older, standard type of heparin has been used extensively in pregnancy, for prolonged periods and for various indications, with no fetal problems. Less data is available about newer formulations (called low molecular weight heparin), although they are being used in pregnancy more and more, and we know that they also do not cross the placenta. All indications are that they are equally safe and they are rapidly becoming the drugs of choice.

Given the increased risk of thromboembolism in pregnancy, it is surprising that it is not standard practice to take specific preventive measures during and after cesarean section. I feel that employing either pneumatic compression, or heparin for postcesarean prophylaxis (prevention) should be considered for all cesarean patients. We know it is effective, and since we know these patients have an elevated risk for thrombosis, it makes no sense not to consider it. My personal practice is to use pneumatic compression in low-risk patients, and heparin in higher-risk patients for all cesareans. The decision to employ heparin is taken after discussion with the anesthetist, since the timing of the heparin as well as the type of heparin given might be influenced by the anesthetic. Unfortunately, as with all things in medicine, there are possible risks, among which are bleeding complications. With the new low molecular weight heparin this risk seems to be reduced, except for a recognized risk for spinal hematomas. They should only be started about twenty-four hours postspinal, with standard heparin in the interim. Patients are also urged to get up as soon as possible after their operation, and to mobilize as soon as possible. The use of spinal anesthesia helps in this regard, especially if a long-acting opioid (like morphine) is added. The resultant decrease in pain for the first twenty-four hours helps to get patients out of bed and moving. Better and deeper breathing as a result of decreased pain helps significantly to increase effective blood flow from the lower body to the chest and heart from where it is again circulated.

Bleeding

Another of the possible major complications during or after a cesarean section is that of hemorrhage. The average blood loss during routine cesareans is usually estimated at around 1.5 to 2 pints (700 milliliters to one liter). In the normal nonpregnant patient, this would be a significant percentage of total blood volume. The pregnant woman, however, has significant physiological adaptations protecting her against complications of significant blood loss. Normal vaginal delivery causes an average loss of around 500 milliliters (half a liter or just over one pint) of blood with usually no negative effect. The reason that pregnant women can withstand the loss of this amount of blood without suffering the usual consequences is that the hormones of pregnancy have caused a significant increase in blood volume. This increase is around 40 percent of total blood volume. Another adaptation is a greater, percentage-wise increase in blood plasma over the red blood cell number. As a result, for any given volume of blood the pregnant woman has fewer red blood cells than the nonpregnant woman, even though she has an increased number in total. The loss of a certain volume of blood thus leads to the loss of fewer cells than would have occurred without this dilutional effect.

Postpartum bleeding most commonly occurs as a result of a relaxing uterus. This is as true for a postcesarean patient as for one who has had a vaginal delivery. During pregnancy the blood flow through the uterus, which supplies the nutrients and oxygen to the placenta and to the fetus, is incredible. Almost the whole blood volume of the pregnant woman at term (toward the end of pregnancy) circulates through her uterus every few minutes. This blood flows through open vascular canals to the placenta and then back into the mother's circulation. After separation of the placenta from the uterus, it is imperative that the flow be cut off almost instantaneously to prevent otherwise inevitable death in a few short minutes. Anyone who has ever bled from a wound (and that probably includes everybody) will agree that the normal way that bleeding stops in a wound will not suffice. The normal clotting mechanisms, which come into play to slow bleeding under these conditions, are far too slow. It is indeed true that nature has devised an ingenious way to stop the bleeding from the postpartum uterus, almost like turning off a tap.

The uterine muscles form an intricate network of muscle fibers weaving their way around the blood vessels and channels. Contractions of the uterus have the ability to cut off bleeding by instantaneously restricting thin-walled channels. During labor, this safety mechanism can sometimes cause problems with decreased blood flow to the fetus. As a mechanism to stop the postpartum bleeding, however, it is an effective and absolutely crucial occurrence. Any relaxation of the uterus after delivery usually leads to bleeding. Unfortunately, the uterus is somewhat more prone to relaxing after cesarean than after normal delivery. Obstetricians are very aware of this fact and will usually take adequate precautions. The risk of relaxation of the uterus (also called uterine atony) is also significantly reduced after elective cesarean than after a cesarean performed after many hours of obstructed labor, where the uterus is simply worn out.

Although the blood loss during cesarean section can be double what is lost during normal vaginal delivery, it is usually not clinically important and blood transfusion is rarely necessary.

Any patient with bleeding disorders, or with medical or obstetrical conditions that make dangerous bleeding more likely, should obviously be carefully counseled and informed, and might not be a candidate for elective cesarean. It also stands to reason that a woman contemplating cesarean should be in the best medical condition possible, and that obviously must include the absence of preventable anemia (abnormally low blood count, usually related to lack of iron).

SURGICAL INJURIES

Most surgical procedures carry an inherent risk of injuries to organs not directly involved in the surgery; cesarean is no exception. Injuries to the bowel, bladder, ureters, and blood vessels have all been described. Fortunately, these injuries are rare. The most common injury is to the bladder. This usually occurs either upon entering the abdominal cavity, or when freeing the bladder from the lower segment of the uterus. Fortunately these injuries are usually very easily dealt with via simple sutures and by keeping the bladder empty with a catheter. Injuries to the bowel or ureters could potentially be more serious, especially if overlooked.

I firmly believe that the incidence of injuries during elective cesarean will be found to be lower than during emergency cesarean. This makes logical sense in that an elective cesarean is, by definition, a more relaxed procedure usually performed with less haste. The fetal head is usually higher in the pelvis and not wedged tightly and deeply into the pelvis as in so many cases where cesareans are performed during labor. Injuries often occur in the process of delivering such wedged babies. In such cases it is often necessary for someone to push the baby's head up from the vaginal side, since the head might be so tightly wedged in the pelvis, that it might be impossible to get either a hand or a forceps blade around the head from above. Since the vagina is not sterile, it can easily be seen how such maneuvers during emergency cesarean can further increase the infection rate.

A repeat cesarean, exactly like a repeat abdominal operation for any other reason, is technically somewhat more difficult and carries a slightly higher risk for complications. Usually this is not a problem, however. A good surgical technique and meticulous care during the performance of the surgery will minimize the potential risk. Although this risk can never be zero, even in the best hands, incidental injuries during cesareans really are very uncommon. The risk of significant adhesions increase with number of cesareans, and indeed with the number of any abdominal surgeries. I'd say that three cesareans is, in my mind, the number after which I feel distinctly uncomfortable recommending further pregnancies. Having said that, I remember a colleague in British Columbia doing cesarean number eight on a woman. Persisting to get pregnant after having multiple previous cesareans is NOT recommended! Elective primary cesarean would NOT be a reasonable option for women who could be expected to have more than three children.

Psychological Problems, Bonding Problems, and Postpartum Depression

I have mentioned previously that it seems as if there might be an increased incidence of depression or maladaptation and abnormal bonding with the baby after cesarean. I strongly believe, however, that seeing this merely as a complication of cesarean section is a simplistic generalization and is wrong. Some of my most ecstatic and well-adapted patients and new mothers had their babies by cesarean birth.

There are many factors that could play a role in this regard and, of course, every patient's expectations are different. The reaction of any specific patient cannot be known beforehand, but I do believe there are a few general truths. Any patient that has been brainwashed into believing that vaginal birth is the only acceptable way to have a baby, and that any other way would indicate a failure of herself as a woman and a mother, can be expected to be upset, disappointed, or even pathologically depressed after having undergone a cesarean section. By comparison, it follows that the woman who has considered all her options carefully and who has come to the conclusion that cesarean birth would be best is certainly less likely to have these emotional problems. To expect increased emotional difficulty after cesarean simply related to the mode of delivery is thus simplistic and may become a self-fulfilling prophecy. It all revolves around expectations, beliefs, and even peer pressure.

The birth of a baby, in itself, is such an emotional and overwhelming occurrence that the route of delivery is of lesser importance. No one can deny, however, that the feeling of accomplishment after the vaginal delivery of a baby after labor will be lacking in cesarean births. This feeling can sometimes be an almost overwhelmingly positive sensation that reaffirms the woman's strength, womanhood, and ability to bring to a conclusion this most important biological aspect of being a woman. It is thus possible that even the well-informed and well-prepared woman delivered by cesarean, might feel some regret later on. This is one of the important reasons

I believe that the decision to have an elective cesarean birth should only be taken after a process of discussion, and evaluation of the facts and risks. The patient's own specific emotional needs should not be neglected and, as I have stressed before, this is *not* a decision that should be made during labor.

Intra-abdominal Adhesions

Any abdominal surgery can potentially lead to adhesion formation inside the abdominal cavity and cesarean section is no exception. These adhesions sometimes present soon after the surgery with symptoms of bowel obstruction, but the more common scenario is that of delayed presentation at a time remote from that of the surgery. These adhesions can also present with abdominal pain when they interfere with other organs, but the most common presentation by far is acute or subacute (partial) bowel obstruction. Further surgery is then indicated, often as an emergency procedure, which can then lead to an exacerbation of the adhesion formation process.

Fortunately, cesarean sections do not often lead to adhesions causing bowel obstruction. Although adhesions are not uncommon, they more frequently occur in front of the uterus and most commonly involve the bladder. The most likely clinical significance of postcesarean adhesions is that they could make the next cesarean more difficult and as a result increase the probability of operative complications, especially bladder injuries. This is one of the reasons that the risks of elective cesarean will probably outweigh the benefits in women planning many (more than three) children. Adhesions from previous major abdominal surgery could potentially interfere with the function of the fallopian tubes and thus lead to infertility problems. This is a particularly unlikely complication of an uncomplicated cesarean section, however.

Placenta Accreta and Placenta Previa

Placenta accreta is a condition that fortunately is quite rare, since it can have devastating consequences for the future reproductive career of a woman and can cause one of the most serious obstetrical emergencies, usually immediately after childbirth. It should be noted that I stress "childbirth" and not "cesarean birth." This problem is not exclusive to cesarean but is a potential complication of any birth. Most cases occur after vaginal delivery but that is probably true because most births are vaginal.

Placenta accreta literally means, "stuck placenta." This occurs if the placenta is abnormally attached to the uterine wall with the result that it cannot release after childbirth. The results can be dramatic with severe hemorrhage being the possible result of attempting to remove the placenta. A hysterectomy is sometimes the only way to deal with the situation.

Cesarean increases the risk of placenta accreta, especially if the placenta is low lying in the general area of the previous uterine incision.

"Placenta previa," means a placenta is in front of the birth canal opening. In practical terms this means that the placenta is blocking the inner cervix, blocking the baby's birth route. Partial placenta previas are often detected by an early ultrasound. When the lower segment of the uterus is lower than the placenta, later ultrasounds usually find a significantly reduced number of placenta previas. However, a more complete covering of the cervix by the placenta is unlikely to resolve. The underlying problem is an implantation of the placenta in an abnormally low position in the uterus. In the case of a previous cesarean section, the finding of placenta previa, especially if the placenta is located toward the anterior (front) part of the uterus, raises concern of a placenta accreta. It is thought that the scar formation leads to an abnormal placental attachment. In these cases, the placenta in fact grows into the wall of the uterus with the resultant failure of the detachment mechanisms after birth. Attempts to remove it might only cause its piecemeal removal, with heavy bleeding as the result. As mentioned, emergency surgery is sometimes necessary.

Although the incidence of placenta accreta is higher after previous cesarean births, the actual overall incidence is low. Ultrasound exclusion of a low-lying placenta over the anterior part of the lower segment (thus directly underlying the previous cesarean scar) makes it very unlikely indeed.

Amniotic and Air Embolism

These are rare but potentially fatal complications of any pregnancy. The incidence may be slightly increased during cesarean section. Suturing the uterus inside the body cavity, without delivering the uterus through the wound, might minimize the risk. An explanation of these problems is outside the scope of this book.

Abruptio Placentae

An abruptio placentae occurs when the placenta tears away from the side of the uterus. Since the placenta is the life-support system of the fetus, such a development may have serious consequences. A serious abruption can lead to fetal distress and even death. Abruptio can also lead to maternal bleeding, and could be a potentially serious complication for the mother as well.

Increased risk of abruption after cesarean is not a well-established fact. I found only one study that found this (as a doubling in risk), and in my mind the real significance of this is still open to future clarification.

Rupture of the Uterine Scar

Having a cesarean section significantly impacts on future pregnancies. Not only is there the small possibility of increased risk of difficulties getting pregnant, but the subsequent pregnancies also are impacted. Some of these have already been mentioned, for instance the increased risk of placenta accreta. In addition, the uterus has a scar where it was previously incised. This scar, like most other scars, is not as strong as the rest of the intact uterus, and as a result constitutes a weak area in the integrity of the uterus. During pregnancy this is not usually a problem as the intra-uterine pressure is unlikely to become significant enough to put the integrity of the scar at risk. During labor, however, there is a risk of scar dehiscence (pulling apart slowly) or a sudden rupture of the scar. This sounds scary, and indeed it might be a catastrophic occurrence. In the best-case scenario, such a dehiscence or imminent rupture during labor will be noticed and immediate cesarean section will be performed. For this reason, most hospitals doing VBAC, also called "trial of scar," insist on an intravenous infusion, as well as continuous electronic monitoring, with one-on-one nursing care at all times. Cesarean section should be able to be performed within ten to fifteen minutes. This is one of the biggest problems since many rural and smaller hospitals without twenty-four-hour, in-house staff and immediate operating room access simply cannot guarantee that.

The reason that these patients are considered high risk in labor is that the clinical rupture rate is significant. The overall rate is considered to be about 0.7 percent, but the incidence depends on many factors, and a few studies have found a much higher overall rate. If the labor is within two years from the preceding cesarean, and the uterine incision was closed in only one layer during the cesarean, the risk increases to 5 percent, clearly a rate that would make most people uncomfortable. The rupture rate is also increased after more than one previous cesarean section.

If the rupture involves the whole incision, the baby or the placenta might be pushed out into the abdominal cavity through the force of the contractions. Severe bleeding might also ensue, putting both mother and baby at immediate risk. Fetal death, brain damage, and other severe long-term negative fetal complications are possible. The traumatic nature of the rupture could cause a tear in the maternal bladder, causing significant difficulty in fixing the bladder. The damage, as well as the bleeding, could lead to the need to perform a hysterectomy.

Having discussed all of these negative and scary things, I should emphasize that VBAC is successful and uncomplicated in up to 65 or 70 percent of women. The rest end up with an emergency cesarean, often after many hours of labor. This is the worst possible outcome in terms of delivery (other than some acute event), since emergency cesarean after "trial of scar" labor is associated with significantly higher complication rates than either successful VBAC or elective cesarean birth.

Most ruptures are not as dramatic as what has been described. Commonly one notices certain pointers that indicate an increased risk, or the beginning of a slow rupture or dehiscence, and one can take the appropriate action (cesarean). In light of this, most obstetrical societies in the world encourage VBAC, provided the rules are followed and there are no contraindications.

The risk of scar rupture after classical cesarean section is totally different. After a classical cesarean it is unwise to attempt vaginal delivery, and cesarean is the only option. A classical cesarean is where the incision in the uterus is made longitudinally (up and down) instead of transverse (horizontal). Where the transverse incision of the more common cesarean involves the lower segment of the uterus, the incision of a classical cesarean involves the higher, thicker body of the uterus. Since this is the area of the uterus where the maximal muscle effort is situated during labor, it is more likely to tear the scar, in which case a catastrophe is all but assured. Classical cesarean is not routinely done today, except in certain exceptional circumstances, for instance extreme premature birth.

It should be obvious then that the decision to have an elective cesarean birth should not be taken lightly. That decision should only be made with the realization that it will impact on all future reproductive decisions and events.

Neonatal Complications of Cesarean Section

The question about what the fetus would choose is quite complicated. It is well known that a number of healthy and normal fetuses die intrauterine after having reached viability (adequate development to survive outside the uterus). The saddest thing obstetricians sometimes have to do is to make a diagnosis of an intrauterine death at term. This happens in a certain percentage of women, although thankfully it is low. Even so, it is currently one of the most common causes of perinatal mortality in the developed world. It is devastating to diagnose a fetal death in a situation where you know that if the baby had been born just a day earlier, it would have presumably been perfectly healthy. Often no cause of the death can be found. In 1985, Feldman and Freiman calculated in a controversial paper that between 36 and 360 such fetuses could be saved for every extra maternal death that would have resulted from doing universal cesarean sections at maturity. Since many of these deaths occur during the last few weeks of pregnancy, elective cesarean would prevent many of these occurrences.

More recent studies and surveys have shown clearly that the risks to the fetus due to vaginal delivery are orders of magnitude greater than many other activities where our society often institutes precautionary measures. I'm thinking here of riding a motorcycle without a helmet, drinking and driving, and the like. Dr. Nicholas Fisk (an obstetrician from London) recently made the following statement at a conference I attended in Toronto where he was one of the keynote speakers: "In spite of these risks, and in contrast to many other activities that are illegal because of the risks, vaginal delivery remains (for the time being), legal." In this vein, the American Urogynecologic Society had on the front page of their winter 2003 quarterly report an article entitled: "Informed Concent for Vaginal Delivery."

Cesarean section prevents the potential for complications like fetal distress and intrapartum death from hypoxia (not getting enough oxygen), as well as fetal injuries that sometimes occur as a result of shoulder dystocia (where the shoulders get stuck after the fetal head is delivered). This is a totally unpredictable, and extremely serious, delivery complication.

Vaginal delivery does confer certain advantages, especially in terms of respiratory function. Elective cesarean is associated with an increase in *transient* tachypnoea (increased rate of breathing) and respiratory distress of the newborn. This risk is significantly dependent upon the gestation of the fetus, and the risk drops significantly toward the due date. At thirty-nine weeks the risk of this is less than 2 percent. Most of these problems are as the name indicates, transient.

There is some evidence that babies born by elective cesarean section have lower stress scores as measured by crying. Those born by operative vaginal deliveries had the highest stress scores.[4] It is interesting to note that adults prone to violent suicide were more likely to have had a traumatic delivery, for instance an instrumental vaginal delivery.[5]

Effects of Cesarean Birth on the Newborn

One of the worst things that could happen during elective cesarean birth is if the baby is delivered prematurely. The most serious risk of premature birth is undeveloped lungs, causing respiratory problems or even failure. Fortunately, modern ultrasound technology makes gestational age determination very accurate, so this problem should not be of great concern. The ultrasound should be done as early as possible, certainly before twenty-two weeks, since ultrasounds after this date cannot determine accurate gestational age.

Most women are aware of the methods of gestational age determination according to the last menstrual date. Even though this method can be quite accurate, given certain preconditions, large studies have shown that, on average, ultrasound determination is more accurate and is preferable if an elective cesarean section is to be planned. The reason for this is that ovulation is sometimes delayed, with fertilization and the start of the pregnancy thus being delayed up to two weeks. If preceding menstrual cycles were not completely regular the uncertainty is compounded immensely. For these and other reasons it is preferable to use the ultrasound for dating. The cesarean should be planned for after the thirty-eighth week of gestation, when it is almost certain that the infant's lungs and other critical organ systems have adequately developed.

Even if great care is taken to determine gestational age accurately and to perform the cesarean section only after thirty-eight weeks (by definition, a full term pregnancy), respiratory difficulties are more common in cesarean-born infants than vaginally born ones. These difficulties are usually transient and of little consequence, but they do cause a higher percentage of cesarean-born infants to spend time in an incubator. The reason is the absence of the natural squeezing that vaginally born infants experience during their long passage through the vaginal birth canal. In the uterus the infant's lungs are filled with amniotic fluid that the unborn baby breathes in and out constantly since very early in the pregnancy. This breathing action and the presence of amniotic fluid is absolutely essential for normal lung development. During birth, the squeezing through the birth passage causes an increased pressure inside the infant's chest. This increased pressure causes the fluid to be taken up by the blood vessels and lymphatic channels (channels similar to veins but filled with excess fluid) in the chest and lungs, thereby emptying the lung airspaces of the fluid to a large degree. Some of it might also be squeezed out through the infant's mouth. It is obvious that these processes do not occur during cesarean birth. Undeveloped lungs in the inadvertently prematurely cesarean-born infant will exacerbate this problem and can lead to significant respiratory difficulties. Fortunately however, in the full-term cesarean-born, the increased lung fluid usually leads to a very temporary condition called, appropriately, "wet lung." The most common situation is that the fluid gets reabsorbed within a few seconds to minutes after birth with no further consequences.

A far more serious problem is a condition called "meconium aspiration." This is where an unborn infant moves its bowels inside the uterus and then inhales the meconium (unborn baby poop). Meconium is formed from sterile material, mainly cells that have sloughed from the developing fetus's immature bowel, and should not be confused with feces. Be that as it may, it is still very bad news if inhaled by any fetus since it has the potential to cause serious harm or even death. A common reason for fetuses to pass meconium while still in the uterus is stress, often during the birth process. Fetuses also often pass meconium even before labor initiates however, especially in the post-term (gestational length significantly longer than the average of forty weeks) or growth-retarded fetus. Cesarean sections could be expected, therefore, to prevent some cases of meconium aspiration since it will be done at thirty-eight weeks and the stress of labor is eliminated. If the fetus has already passed meconium in the uterus, for whatever reason, and if aspirated (inhaled), the risk of potentially serious meconium aspiration syndrome is elevated. The squeeze-related emptying of the infant's lungs is absent, and the presence of meconium in conjunction with "wet lung syndrome," can cause serious trouble.

My own firstborn, by cesarean (not elective) at forty-two weeks, spent three days in a neonatal intensive care unit with serious meconium aspiration syndrome. So I do have firsthand, traumatic experience with this problem. Although her situation was completely different than the baby born by purely elective cesarean in an otherwise normal pregnancy at thirty-eight to forty weeks, respiratory problems should never be underestimated.

During the cesarean, most obstetricians and/or pediatricians (depending on the local custom) will, in a case where meconium is found, suction the infant's mouth and nose passages as soon as the baby's head is delivered through the wound. This will minimize the risk of the infant inhaling the meconium with the first breath.

Convalescence After Cesarean Birth

The women that take the longest to recover after delivery are those who undergo emergency cesarean section after a long, arduous but ultimately unsuccessful vaginal delivery attempt. It stands to reason that these women are not only physically and emotionally exhausted, but they are also often depressed, or at least disappointed, and have suffered a severe knock to their self-confidence. They probably haven't eaten for a long time, and might be dehydrated. Their risk for, and the resultant recurrence of, problems like wound infections, is elevated.

By contrast, the women who have elective cesareans arrive at the hospital about an hour before the scheduled procedure. Although apprehensive, the patient is refreshed and she knows what to expect, and exactly what is going to happen. She *knows* she is not going to suffer. She has full confidence that her baby is going to be born in excellent condition. About three hours after having arrived at the hospital, she is in the postpartum ward with her baby in her arms. Although she can't eat immediately, she can take sips of water, and can eat that evening. She starts walking around that afternoon, since the spinal epimorphine that the anesthetist gave keeps her mostly pain free for up to eighteen hours. Most of my cesarean patients go home on day three or four after cesarean. Most vaginal delivery patients go home on day two.

Most vaginal birth patients have at least a second-degree vaginal tear that causes significant discomfort initially, and can be uncomfortable for months. It can also potentially cause dyspareunia (painful sex).

Minor morbidity (complications) for a few weeks after delivery is common irrespective of the method of delivery. But those that had assisted vaginal delivery, and specifically forceps delivery, could experience persistent problems for months, and if significant pelvic floor damage was sustained, these problems could persist for a lifetime.

Notes

1. B. P. Sachs, J. Yeh, et al., "Cesarean Section-Related Maternal Mortality in Massachusetts, 1954-1985," *Obstetrics and Gynecology* 71 (1988): 385–88.

2. M. E. Hannah, W. J. Hannah, S. A. Hewson, et al., "Planned Cesarean Section versus Planned Vaginal Birth for Breech Presentation at Term: A Randomized Multicentre Trial," *Lancet* 356 (2000): 1375–83.

3. D. B. Scott and M. E. Tunstall, "Serious Complications Associated with Epidural/Spinal Blockade in Obstetrics: A Two-Year Prospective Study," *International Journal of Obstetric Anesthesia* 4 (1995): 133–39.

4. A. Taylor and N. M. Fisk, "Mode of Delivery and Subsequent Stress Response," *Lancet* 355, no. 9198 (2000): 120.

5. B. Jacobsen, "Obstetric Care and Proneness of Offspring to Suicide as Adults: Case-Control Study," *British Medical Journal* 317, no. 7169 (1998): 1346–49.

NINETEEN
The Forum

www.pelvicfloor.com

Until this book, there has been little information directed to a lay audience regarding the entire gamut of pelvic floor disorders. Women have had very few places to turn, few people to talk to, and the isolation factor surrounding their symptoms has deepened. Few publishers knew or wanted to know anything at all about the pelvic floor. But after seeing women day after day suffering from a variety of so-called hush-hush maladies, I realized that there had to be a safe place to share feelings, ask questions, and air frustrations. I (M.M.) launched www.pelvicfloor.com in October 2000. An earlier draft of this book (one that focused in larger part on the choice of delivery issue) was posted there, along with a document-and-image library. Most importantly, the site also offers a discussion forum, a place with no faces and few real names but a considerable number of questions, comments, and debate.

From the postings in the forum, participants can view the comments and advice from women who are incredibly knowledgeable about their own medical histories. In many cases, these are women who spend considerable time researching current options and treatments. They can often recite the entire glossary of terms and implications. They are so eager to share this information and so very comforted to know that they are not alone in this battle. There are also a few medical professionals weighing in, some with differing points of view. And, any of my opinions and recommendations posted on the site are mine alone. Since each person's problems are different and should be seen in the context of their whole medical history, any information obtained from the site should be discussed with a personal and responsible medical practitioner before any firm decisions are made. However, the site is intended to arm women with the necessary knowledge, empowering them to take a more personal, proactive charge of their health.

There are literally hundreds of postings and responses archived on the site since its inception. In total, they comprise an entire book-length project unto themselves. With that said, we'd like to share a few standout excerpts that illustrate the poignant need for ongoing discussion and research in the field of pelvic health.

On Cesarean Section After a Vaginal Delivery

Wary: I had a very simple vaginal labor at the age of forty, a seven-pound boy, and no real problems, but did suffer a grade-two tear. I did beg to have a cesarean section at the beginning of my pregnancy but was really pressured into having a vaginal delivery. I could not recover well, went to a urogynecologist and found that I had a cystocele. It appears that my history of chronic constipation, plus twenty years of playing a wind instrument four to five hours a day (equal to weight lifting) created some laxity in the ligaments which, along with the stress and stretching of vaginal delivery, led to the cystocele. Luckily I recovered most pelvic muscle strength with muscle training and biofeedback, and have only occasional stress incontinence. I do my "Kegels" religiously and now, ten months later, I am almost back to normal—but I can no longer jog or exercise as strenuously as before.

I am considering having another child. The urogynecologist certainly believes I would be a candidate for a cesarean section. However, of the several fine obstetricians I have consulted, most feel that any damage was really done with the first child and that a cesarean may just damage other areas. Also they feel that the damage may have been done during pregnancy itself, not just during labor.

I am extremely wary of another vaginal delivery. In fact, I would almost consider not having another child because of my fear of another vaginal delivery (I could not walk for one month and had to stop my musical career for several more months). So, with all the talk of vaginal delivery after cesarean, what about the reverse?

Dr. Murphy: Very interesting question and unfortunately there is no right and no wrong answer. It certainly appears as if a significant percentage of damage will be sustained during the first vaginal delivery. However, there is an additional cumulative risk of disorders (apparently, especially anal incontinence) for each subsequent delivery.

One report at the conference (2001 annual conference of the American Urogynecologic Society) by Zetterstron et al. from Sweden found that urinary incontinence is doubled after vaginal delivery, but that the number of subsequent deliveries did not significantly influence the incidence of symptoms over the five years of the study. The incidence of urinary incontinence they found was 23 percent at nine months and 37 percent at five years. Ten percent of women (after vaginal delivery) had both urinary and anal incontinence at nine months and 20 percent at five years.

Of course the incidence of these disorders depends on the definitions used to diagnose them, which is part of the problem when comparing across studies and populations. But the fact is, the incidence is significant.

The question of the influence of pregnancy itself is also interesting. It is becoming clear that pregnancy per se, does have a negative influence on anterior vaginal support specifically, and does lead to some women developing urinary incontinence. The incidence during pregnancy is significant. Many women arrive at the labor units believing their amniotic fluid is leaking, and it is often difficult to persuade them that no, it is actually urine that is leaking.

I think I will be correct to say that most urogynecologists believe that the vaginal birthing process adds further significant stress and often damage to the pelvic integrity.

So, should you have a cesarean or not? Unfortunately I cannot answer that question. My feeling is that you should have a right to decide how YOU would like your baby born. If you decide on a cesarean section, that wish should be respected. Your responsibility is to make yourself aware of the risks of both approaches, and eventually accept whatever complications arise, should any happen. Note that today's litigious society expects perfect outcomes in all situations, and if something goes wrong, it must be somebody's fault. Your doctor doesn't always know what is best, but might only think so. . . .

Less Wary: I will consider my options (although now really leaning toward a cesarean section because I feel my age and history will make a C-section a quicker recovery—and yes things can go wrong either way).

But I greatly appreciate the confidence boost towards allowing women to make educated choices. I also appreciate your clearly written article on "Choosing Cesarean Birth."

Any anger I may have about the results of my first vaginal birth is related to the unbalanced and incredible pressure put on me to choose vaginal birth. My research led me, and my gut reaction at the time, was that I wanted a C-section—but after all, "they" are the experts, so I went against my inclination.

I want to emphasize that I consulted with a total of eight gynecologists in my very large city, and all were adamant about vaginal delivery even though the three women doctors *all* had C-sections. Other women I have spoken to were also pressured to have vaginal births. I do, though, still consider that I made my own decision to have a vaginal birth, and I am aware that most of my friends who had vaginal births did not experience the problems I had.

More trust in my own self-knowledge and more awareness that this is a debated topic within the medical community would have given me more assurance that I wasn't "crazy" or "just afraid of pain" to want a C-section. Your answer made it clear that there are risks involved in either situation. It is too bad that so much litigation also makes doctors unable to do what they think might truly be best in various situations, or to even present the full picture to their patients.

Thoughts from Brazil

I am a thirty-two-year-old doctor and I have been practicing obstetrics after my three-year residency and my university training some ten years ago. Here in Brazil, we have this amazing title of champion as to the cesarean rate—about 80 percent in private hospitals and clinics and about 30 percent and rising in public institutions. It means those that can pay are those that can choose. I've been asking myself why Brazilian women are so different from the rest of the world, or if we are practicing bad obstetrics, and the more I think about it the more I am confused. Even my approach is changing of late. First, I used to insist on a normal delivery because I was really convinced that it was best for my patient. But after some hard labors and disappointed patients who couldn't find paradise in such a painful experience, I was less sure about my convictions. Although I still have a strange "guilty" feeling of failure after a C-section.

I certainly feel that a C-section rate of 80 percent is not reasonable. Many women, I believe, are really manipulated by their doctors. What would you do if the doctor says your baby could be in a dangerous situation? But can I choose the way a woman will undertake this important event? Can I assert that it will be a pleasant and wonderful moment? Is pain the way of achieving something? No women accept pain and suffering like normal things anymore. But this is such a new concern!

I hope that we can discuss this important subject all over the world with different cultures.

A Differing Point of View

Outraged: I am frankly outraged by your site! I have many differing opinions and a *man* of your lack of experience with having a female pelvis would never be able to fully understand a *woman's* pelvis. I have been side by side with women for the past ten years experiencing nontraumatic vaginal birth, traumatic birth, and cesarean section. Obviously you have not spent time with a new mother through the initial postoperative phase and do not understand the magnitude of ripping an infant from an abdomen. I strongly differ on your OPINION that natural childbirth advocates do not experience dealing with women with severe urinary incontinence, diminished sex lives, inhibited physical activity, and loss of quality of life. I, for one, pushed for four hours and delivered a ten-pound baby many years ago. Had I been mutilated as you propose, I would be experiencing all of the above!

In addition, your conclusion that there is no effective way to predict these perineal outcomes is also misspoken. There is extensive research to show that the act of inflicting episiotomies, not educating women to strengthen the perineum before and after childbirth, and physicians interrupting childbirth with unnecessary interventions are the actual causes. Please get current, get real, and get out of the profession of needlessly scaring women.

Dr. Murphy: I honestly thank you for expressing your sincerely held opinion, which of course has some merit. I do want to point out, though, the word of caution that I post on the Web site: The manuscript on the right to choose a cesarean birth was written to be controversial and to stimulate debate. Keep that in mind when reading it! Conclusions and opinions expressed are mine alone, and I can't stress enough the need for building a trusting relationship with your own physician. Read my thoughts, think for yourself, and then discuss it with your doctor.

I would also like to ask you to go to the bulletin board of the Web site and read the advice I have given so far. Also read the *entire* manuscript and not just a few selected chapters. Then write back to me. I have a suspicion that your very harsh opinion will have changed, even though we might still completely disagree about many things. The comments you made indicate that you have not yet done the above, since (just for example) I indeed discuss episiotomy and pelvic floor exercises in great detail, and encourage pelvic floor strengthening repetitively.

My aim is simply that of empowerment by knowledge, and it's certainly not that all women should have cesarean births, but rather that they should be educated about the pelvic floor and the possible negative effects of childbirth. It is my belief that choosing a cesarean birth should be a valid choice based on complete informed consent and knowledge of benefits versus risks. But in the end, it should be a completely personal decision. Keeping this information from women (as it seems you would prefer) is in my opinion paternalistic, disrespectful, and disempowering to women.

Although I am one of only a few expressing these views in a public forum (and thus should expect to be a bit of a lightning rod), they are commonly discussed at obstetrical, and especially urogynecological meetings. Since childbirth is an emotional issue, one could expect many strongly held viewpoints, but I believe we should at least try to differ from each other without resorting to sexist comments. Thanks again for taking the time to send me your comments.

Anna responds to the previous discussion: I wasn't going to post again until I had useful data to report but this inane post from "outraged" forces me to respond. To claim there is no place for C-sections is ignorance. Perhaps your physical configuration permitted delivery of a ten-pound baby, but mine did not.

If I had had a C-section with my last baby, I would have eleven years of my life back. I would not have suffered years of unbearable pelvic and back muscle pain, and nerve pain, which has basically disabled me.

I have not been able to run and play with my sons. In fact, by the time my youngest was eighteen months old, my condition prevented me from even picking him up.

This damage is solely due to a poorly thought out vaginal delivery that should have been a C-section. I believe that rants like this post have led to C-sections not being performed when indicated.

People who make these kinds of rash statements need to understand that simply because they have a passionate belief, it does not make that belief correct.

On Prolapse

Jessica: I am from the U.K. and finally found your site after I searched extensively for information. I am thirty-two, have four children, and I had a hysterectomy in 1999. The last six months or so I have felt a heavy feeling down below. After keeping it to myself for quite some time, I finally decided to take a look with a mirror. I found a large lump that gets worse upon standing up. My doctor examined me and thinks I have a prolapsed vagina. I had my cervix removed; also my womb and they kindly left me with my ovaries. At thirty-two, I feel like such a freak! I feel too young to have to worry about such things. I have no sex drive. I'm also very conscious of it when I do try to make love to my husband. In addition, I have backaches, constipation, and urinate often.

Dr. Murphy: Unfortunately it sounds like you might have a vaginal vault prolapse. I cannot make a diagnosis but what you describe would be consistent with such a diagnosis. It basically means that the uppermost part of your vagina has lost its support and is hanging low, which explains why it increases when standing (gravity!). This is why it is so important for doctors to examine patients with these symptoms in the supine (on their back), as well as erect, especially if things don't appear to be consistent with the symptoms in the flat position, or the extent of the problem might be missed.

If you do have this problem, exercises are not going to be of any direct benefit (Kegels or otherwise). You will need surgery. The pessary option is not a viable or long-term option for a young woman.

The surgery usually done first is some sort of vaginal repair and suspension. There are different procedures that could be done and you will have to discuss those with your chosen gynecological surgeon. The results are most often excellent. You should look forward to having it fixed and restoring your function in that area.

TWENTY
Another Perspective

Sarah is fourteen years old and she lives in a village within a country that offers rudimentary health care and no education to speak of, especially not for women. She got married a few months ago. She is her husband's third wife and is expected to bear him many strong sons. After all, sons are the old-age security of any man.

Sarah became pregnant almost immediately, her small thin body straining with the stress of nurturing the growing fetus. When she went into labor, the only care she received was from the witch doctor who examined her with filthy hands and much casting of bones, accompanied by chants and singing.

After thirty-six hours, she had not yet delivered. Already she had pushed for five hours and was tiring fast. Her small pelvis was too small to let the baby through. A lack of nutrition and her young age had seen to that. Ten hours after full dilatation, she had developed a fever and was slowly dehydrating. The nearest hospital was only a few hours by truck, over a bumpy dirt road. But there was no truck, and no ambulance. Eighteen hours later she arrived at the hospital on a donkey's back. She was near death. The baby had died many hours before.

The doctor performed a decompressive procedure on the baby. In essence, the baby's skull was perforated and the brain partially sucked out so that the skull could collapse. In any event, the fetus was finally born. Everybody was relieved. Her fever responded to the antibiotics. She was one of the lucky ones.

When she returned to her village a few days later, she noticed it for the first time—a dripping and wetness when she walked or stood. Soon the dripping became a constant leakage. It wouldn't stop. And the smell . . . she smelled of urine all the time, sitting in it, sleeping in it. Her clothes were always wet and a streak of urine fell behind her as she walked. People began to talk about her, turning their faces from her, avoiding her. Her husband didn't want to talk to her. He eventually kicked her out of the communal hut into a nearby hut where she remained alone.

Then an even more terrible thing started to happen. Feces literally began leaking from her vagina, and there was nothing that would take away the smell.

At that point her husband and the other villagers could no longer tolerate her. She was sent away as she had become a burden too difficult to bear. Her husband could always get another wife.

Where does she go? How can she survive? She can't even turn to prostitution to support herself. She is truly in the most wretched of circumstances.

Although Sarah is a fictional character, sadly her fate is that of thousands of women in Africa and throughout the Third World *today*. Sarah's story was shown in a video at a recent medical conference. I share it without guilt as I feel that if even one person donates money to aid in Third-World maternity care, it will be of great value.

Yes, most of us are saturated with bad-news stories coming from the so-called *Third World*. It used to be easy to ignore them. Recent world events have changed that. We know that it's really not another world, just a different one. We know now that most everything is really a global event. We know now that all people really have the same wishes, yearnings, and fears.

Sometimes it's important to see the bigger world, so that things can be viewed in perspective. In many countries classified as "Third World," medical care is rudimentary, or often even nonexistent, while the rest of us complain about waiting lists, doctors being late, or not getting that epidural immediately. Whereas in the developed world we're debating the relative merits of elective preventative cesarean sections and various high-tech diagnostic and therapeutic options, many Third-World women lack even the most basic health care. While women's health has been a black sheep of health care even in Western countries, in many developing ones, it is practically nonexistent. The results include hundreds of thousands of destroyed lives and mortality figures that are so shocking they are incomprehensible.

I lived in Africa for most of my life. Granted, I lived the same lifestyle that most Western people will recognize as middle class. But I did see real poverty, not the imagined poverty of people living below the "poverty line" in rich countries. Some of the proudest people I've had the privilege to meet were nomadic tribes people in northwestern Namibia. In worldly assets, they would own only a few head of (usually emaciated) cattle. However, they had a certain kind of wealth that is hard to initially understand.

It's a sad fact that increasing contact with Western civilization has made them attuned to their poverty in earthly terms, leading to a breakdown in cultural wealth and dignity, and having disastrous consequences.

I've seen the effect of a lack of Western health care availability, and it is often mirrored in the culture. Many children die early, so it is important to have as many as possible. To do that, many wives are better than one. Children are the only old-age security and pension plan, so the lack of children guarantees suffering. Since many wives die in childbirth, and since some may be barren, the more wives the better. If any wife cannot bear children for whatever reason or fulfill their primary sexual role, they are often ostracized, ridiculed, outcast, and even disowned. In some African countries, proven child-bearing capacity increases a woman's value, and so "out-of-wedlock" children are common ways to first "test" a woman's value as a wife. Of course, the increased "value" will increase the dowry payable to the woman's father.

Many African societies are fiercely chauvinistic. Some of the mentioned sexual beliefs are totally incomprehensible to Western ears, but most are understandable if seen in the context of the world in which it developed. That world did not include (and unfortunately in many cases still doesn't include) Westernized standards of medical care, which leads to the demographic and social consequences to which I allude. The world is seen for what it is: mostly hard and uncompromising to individual wishes and fears. As an individual you are nothing, and probably quickly dead. Security is in numbers, and that means many children. Groups of wives look after their husband, but also after each other, and the communal children.

The point of this discussion is to show how much the loss of the sexual and childbearing function would devastate a woman in such societies. They themselves know nothing else. They are uniformly uneducated and illiterate in what we would understand as "educated," meaning that they have no ability or wish to change their cultures. They want to actualize themselves in their culture, and that means having children. Destruction of this culture by Western influences can only be condoned if something better is put in its place, and in my opinion, a large part of that involves adequate health care.

Unfortunately, Westernization has brought a lot of ills with the good, and for some the good has not arrived at all. The traditional tribal culture has been replaced by a hodge-podge of traditional and Western ways of life in many countries. In some cases, this has led to a breakdown in some of the traditional safeguards and tribal security systems, leaving many people to fend for themselves in a world that is still uncompromising and deaf to individual suffering.

Like the story of Sarah, the real tragedies are single destitute women, those without education to enable them to integrate into the Western world, and those who have lost their sexual and fertility functions. Having no ability to fit in anywhere and no possibility to gain any improvement in their lot, they are doomed.

There is some hope though. Various organizations are actively involved in setting up programs and building hospitals to care for these women. However, the need is so great that the efforts look like drops in the ocean.

So as we continue to debate the pelvic floor issues in *our* world (and so we should), we should spare some thoughts (and maybe more), for our less fortunate fellow humans that share our planet, and our lifetime. In any event, it's always enlightening to see another perspective.

Note: Programs to assist in Third-World maternity healthcare can be found at www.wfmic.org/hidden_ epidemic.htm and www.sogc.org/intl/.

TWENTY-ONE
The Rest of the Story

We began this book with the story of Suzanne, a forty-four-year-old mother of three children, ages twenty-six, twenty-five, and eight. Her incontinence started just after her thirtieth birthday. At age thirty-six, she had her last child. During the delivery, she felt that something inside was not quite right, but she pushed as hard as she could anyway. She felt something tearing in the front and the back. In the year that followed, her incontinence worsened. She felt that something was literally falling out of her vagina. After being homebound and suffering from a severe bout of the blues, she finally consulted with a gynecologist. It was determined that she had a vaginal prolapse and was in need of a cystocele repair. Her last child was only thirteen months old when she had her first surgery. Years passed, and suddenly all the symptoms were back. In her own words, Suzanne tells the rest of the story . . .

"I knew I was prolapsing again. Only this time my periods were starting to mess up. I would have great heavy, stay-at-home-for-three-days periods, sometimes every two weeks. I consulted with my family doctor and I was referred to a specialist. After a thorough examination, he informed me it would be senseless to do a repair without also performing a hysterectomy. My vaginal walls were so weak that they couldn't continue to hold up the weight of the other organs. I needed my uterus and cervix removed as well as a cystocele/rectocele repair—major surgery.

"I went home and thought about everything for the next twenty-four hours. Then I phoned and scheduled an appointment for the surgery.

"About two months later, my husband and I were waiting for preop assessment at the hospital. Those two months had whipped past with end-of-school functions and preparing my home and my little daughter, now eight years old, for the months ahead.

"On the day of my surgery, my husband and I arrived at the hospital about two and a half hours ahead of time. After getting settled in my room and being prepped—shaved and an IV started—we waited, and waited. Four hours after I was due to go in, the nurse finally came and got me. We traveled a maze of corridors and I was left in the middle of one of them, next to an office. Many people walked back and forth past me, some introducing themselves as nurses, doctors, or the anesthetist who would be assisting in my surgery. Then I saw the surgeon briefly. Very soon I was wheeled into the OR and very soon I was fast asleep. My husband recalls that it was about two and a half hours later that I was wheeled back to my room. Things are pretty hazy about that evening.

"I remember my husband and elder daughter coming to see me the next day, and I was wishing that I wasn't hooked up to the oxygen so that I wouldn't look as bad as I felt. At some point the nurses came in and tried to make me stand, or better, to walk. With two of them assisting me I managed to shuffle sideways about a foot before I was overcome with pain and nausea. Back to bed I went. The rest of day two and day three, I felt really lousy. Apparently my blood count was dropping, so I was closely monitored. Blood was taken often and my temperature was checked. By about noon on Sunday, the doctor decided that I needed to go back to surgery. He suspected that there was an "oozer" somewhere. Sometime that afternoon I once again made the trip through the corridors to the OR. I had already been given a unit of blood and they had another to give me while in surgery. This time there was less waiting, and before I knew it, I was back in my own room with three more tiny incisions in my abdomen. This made a total of five with my first surgery.

"I don't remember much about day four. I guess I probably slept between the times when I was getting my IV meds changed and getting shots of morphine for pain.

"The next morning my catheter came out. What a relief not to have that bag attached and the annoying tube running across my legs. The only problem was, I couldn't urinate on my own. I didn't even have the urge. And before I realized what was happening, my bladder was really full. I went to the bathroom to try to relieve myself, but to no avail. By this time I was in excruciating pain and had to ring for the nurses from the bathroom. I was locked right up and couldn't move. The pain was unlike anything I had ever experienced. After what seemed like an eternity, the nurses got me back to bed and drained my bladder with a catheter. The relief was enormous. So I was ready to try again. About three hours later I was really uncomfortable and nothing I did would make me 'go.' Once again, the nurses came in and set up their catheter tray and relieved the pressure. As luck would have it, the whole procedure had to be repeated a few hours later and once again the catheter was permanently affixed for the night. I felt that I had taken a giant step backward.

"The sixth morning, I laid awake in the semidark. I felt horrible. I couldn't shake the feeling that I had gotten myself into a terrible mess. I had been away from my eight-year-old daughter for a week now, and I had thoughts that I might never see her again. All I wanted to do was hold her and be back on my own property, walking on my grass. I was mad at myself for electing to have this stupid surgery and putting myself in jeopardy. I don't ever remember feeling as depressed as this. I cried to myself, and when the doctor came to see me I told him how horrible I felt and how much I missed my daughter. I was fighting the tears again. By the time my husband arrived, I was a mess and broke down in his arms. The feeling of despair was overwhelming. During the day, I did get up and the catheter was removed again, and some time in the afternoon I did urinate on my own. "That was such a feeling of accomplishment that finally I could see some brightness. My husband spent ten hours at the hospital with me that day. Our wedding vows, "in sickness and in health," sure came into play. He was really my "rock" and I felt truly blessed to have him by my side.

"The next day seemed so much brighter. My bladder was finally functioning on its own, although it was really slow. I still hadn't had a bowel movement and that's the next thing I concentrated on. I had been given stool softeners regularly and I was drinking as much water and prune juice as I could handle. I walked around as much as possible, both inside and outside, and was feeling progressively better emotionally—physically was a bit slower. My IV was removed (I had seven IV sites in all) and I changed rooms. It was my last night in the hospital. The doctor had already told me that if things went well I could be discharged in the morning. Before I went to sleep I got another suppository as well as the stool softeners. Nothing seemed to be working to move my bowels. (It's funny now how absolutely important that was at the time.)

"The morning of my discharge I was really uncomfortable from not being able to have a bowel movement. I ate a small breakfast and went to have a shower. While in the shower I was overcome with an irresistible urge to go to the bathroom so I figured 'what the hell,' and let everything go. The relief was incredible. I cleaned up and proceeded to get dressed and packed to leave. The doctor came to see me and I told him what happened and we both had a bit of a laugh.

"It was wonderful walking to the parking lot to get the truck. We were facing a four-hour drive home but I didn't care. I was free! My euphoria was short-lived. About one and a half hours after we left the hospital I had to go to the bathroom. We found a bathroom at a popular rest area and I locked myself in. My bladder was being really shy and there were also people knocking on the door and wondering aloud if anyone was inside. I abandoned the idea of 'going' there and we found another rest stop about 45 minutes down the road. By this time I was in pain and feeling nauseated. I was able to relieve myself in the highly odorous restroom. I took some Tylenol and we cleared out the backseat so I could lie down. The pain in my bladder was increasing rapidly and I had visions of going back to the hospital although the nearest one was still over an hour away. I finally asked my husband to pull over and he found a lovely, private spot near a river. I was able to relax and squatted near the truck until I could urinate. We spent about thirty minutes in this secluded, peaceful spot until I was confident that I could make the next leg of the journey. I knew now how to get the relief I needed and could enjoy the rest of the trip.

"It's been six weeks since my surgery. I am amazed at how good I feel, but I am reminded constantly that I still need to take it easy. I never want to do this again so I am really cautious. The first couple of weeks at home I was overwhelmed with how absolutely exhausted I got. I sat in the sun on my deck and would get tired and have to lie down. I read a lot of novels and just did nothing. I can still feel the spots where the doctor inserted the mesh tape but I am confident that that will heal as well as everything else has.

"My few words of wisdom: Prepare your body before your surgery. I think a few days prior you should go on a fairly soft diet and drink plenty of fluids. I believe this would have greatly helped my bowel functions.

"Prepare yourself mentally. Know that you are going to feel lousy and weak but that you *will* get over it."

Nobody ever said it would be easy. Nothing in life ever really is. But each of us has the power to make our own choices. There are tradeoffs to almost any choice, but there are also just rewards. Weigh your options carefully and trust that your decision is right for you. Be strong. Do what will benefit *you* in mind and in body. Because the hand that is grabbing yours belongs to the one person who needs you most, as a model, a mentor—and a mother.

APPENDIX A
Resources

ASSOCIATIONS

American College of Obstetricians and Gynecologists (ACOG), 409 12th St., S.W., P.O. Box 96920, Washington, DC 20090-6920, Web site: www.acog.org, E-mail: resources@acog.org. ACOG works primarily in four areas: serving as a strong advocate for quality health care for women, maintaining the highest standards of clinical practice and continuing education for its members, promoting patient education and stimulating patient understanding of and involvement in medical care, and increasing awareness among its members and the public of the changing issues facing women's health care.

American Urogynecologic Society (AUGS), 2025 M St., N.W., Ste. 800, Washington, DC 20036, 202-367-1167, Web site: www.augs.org, E-mail: augs@dc.sba.com. The American Urogynecologic Society, founded in 1979, is dedicated to research and education in urogynecology, and to improved care for women with lower urinary tract disorders.

American Urological Association, Inc. (AUA), 1120 N. Charles St., Baltimore, MD 21201, 410-727-1100, Web site: www.auanet.org, E-mail: aua@auanet.org. Their mission is to foster the highest standards of urologic care by providing a wide range of services including publications, an annual meeting, continuing medical education, and health policy advisory.

Association for Applied Psychophysiology and Biofeedback (AAPB), 10200 W. 44th Ave.; Ste. 304, Wheat Ridge, CO 80033-2840, 303-422-8436, Web site: www.aapb.org, E-mail: aapb@resourcecenter.com. The goals of this association are to promote a new understanding of biofeedback and advance the methods used in this practice. Membership in AAPB is open to professionals interested in the investigation and application of applied psychophysiology and biofeedback, and in the scientific and professional advancement of the field.

International Continence Society (ICS), Southmead Hospital, Bristol BS10 5NB, United Kingdom, 44 117 9503510, Web site: www.icsoffice.org, E-mail: vicky@icsoffice.org. The ICS actively encourages continence promotion throughout the world.

The International Pelvic Pain Society (IPPS), Ste. 402, Women's Medical Plaza, 2006 Brookwood Medical Center Dr., Birmingham, AL 35209, 205-877-2950 or 800-624-9676 if in the United States, Web site: www.pelvicpain.org. The Society wishes to recruit, organize, and educate health care professionals actively involved with the treatment of patients who have chronic pelvic pain. Their goals are to serve as an educational resource for, optimize diagnosis and treatment of, and collate research in chronic pelvic pain.

National Association for Continence (NAFC), P.O. Box 8306, Spartanburg, SC 29305-8306, 800-BLADDER, Web site: www.nafc.org, E-mail: memberservices@nafc.org. NAFC's purpose is to be the leading source for public education and advocacy about the causes, preventions, diagnoses, treatments, and management alternatives for incontinence.

Society of Urologic Nurses and Associates (SUNA), E. Holly Ave., Box 56, Pitman, NJ 08071-0056, 888-TAP-SUNA or 856-256-2335, Web site: www.suna.org. A professional organization committed to excellence in patient care standards and a continuum of quality care, clinical practice, and research through education of its members, patients, families, and community.

Society of Obstetricians and Gynaecologists of Canada (SOGC), 780 Echo Dr., Ottawa, ON, K1S 5R7, Canada, 613-730-4192, 800-561-2416, Web site: www.sogc.medical.org, E-mail: helpdesk@sogc.com. Promotes optimal women's health through leadership, collaboration, education, research, and advocacy in the practice of obstetrics and gynecology.

United Ostomy Association, Inc. (UOA), 19772 MacArthur Blvd., Ste. 200, Irvine, CA 92612-2405, 800-826-0826, Web site: www.uoa.org, E-mail: info@uoa.org. The United Ostomy Association is a volunteer-based health organization dedicated to providing education, information, support, and advocacy for people who have had or will have intestinal or urinary diversions.

Foundations

American Foundation for Urologic Disease (AFUD), 1128 N. Charles St., Baltimore, MD 21201, 410-468-1800, Web site: www.afud.org, E-mail: admin@afud.org. Dedicated to the prevention and cure of urologic disease through the expansion of patient education, public awareness, research, and advocacy.

The Canadian Continence Foundation (CCF), P.O. Box 30, Victoria Branch, Westmount, QC H3Z 2V4, Canada, 514-488-8379, 800-265-9575, Web site: www.continence-fdn.ca, E-mail: help@continence-fdn.ca. The Canadian Continence Foundation enhances the quality of life for people experiencing incontinence by helping patients and their caregivers to confidently seek and access cures and treatment options. To this end, the foundation will implement and encourage important public and professional education, support, advocacy, and research to advance incontinence treatment and/or management.

The June Allyson Foundation, c/o American Urogynecologic Society, 401 N. Michigan Ave., Chicago, IL 60611-4267, 312-644-6610, Web site: www.augs.org/allyson. Promotes, encourages, and financially supports medical research and educational efforts to help advance incontinence care.

National Bladder Foundation (NBF), P.O. Box 1095, Richfield, CT 06877-1095, 877-BLADDER or 203-431-0005, Web site: www.bladder.org, E-mail: debsla@aol.com. NBF promotes the rapid discovery of cures and preventive interventions for the most common bladder diseases through the support of research.

The Simon Foundation for Continence, P.O. Box 835, Wilmette, IL 60091, 800-23-SIMON or 847-864-3913, Web site: www.simonfoundation.org, E-mail: simoninfo@simonfoundation.org. The nonprofit Simon Foundation is dedicated to helping people cope with incontinence by educating them about cure, treatment, and management techniques, while also sensitizing health care professionals to their issues.

Web Sites

About Incontinence, www.aboutincontenence.org

This Web site concentrates on the causes, treatments, and ways of living daily with fecal incontinence.

Agency for Health Care Research and Quality (AHRQ), formerly the Agency for Health Care Policy and Research, www.ahcpr.gov

AHCPR's broad programs of research bring practical, science-based information to medical practitioners and to consumers and other health care purchasers.

Bladder Control Treatments, www.bladder-control-treatments.com

This site focuses on the different types of bladder control treatments available. Treatments are broken down into therapeutic, medical, and surgical intervention. It also recommends supplies and equipment helpful for the comfort and dignity of those with bladder control problems.

CNN Interactive Health, www.cnn.com/HEALTH/

A series of articles related to health issues, hosted by Cable News Network.

Continence Worldwide, www.continenceworldwide.org

The Web site for the Continence Promotion Committee (CPC) of the International Continence Society exists to promote education, services, and public awareness about incontinence throughout the world, and to facilitate communication, exchange of information, and partnerships between continence organizations.

Digital Urology Journal, www.duj.com

A peer-reviewed journal of adult and pediatric urology on the World Wide Web.

Health A to Z, www.healthatoz.com

This medical resource developed by health care professionals includes a suite of Web sites, interactive tools, and projects designed to provide many benefits to the consumer.

Health Canada Online, www.hc-sc.gc.ca/

Federal department responsible for helping Canadians maintain and improve their health.

HeliosHealth.com, www.helioshealth.com

Working closely with physicians, nurse-midwives, and other health professionals, this Web site gives detailed information about specific health topics, access to expert advice from a medical advisory board, and up-to-date health news. There is a discussion forum, hundreds of animations and videos, and an e-mail newsletter. Content is updated daily to give you all of the latest news and research.

InContiNet, www.incontinet.com

An incontinence-focused bulletin board service open to any and all contributors.

Incontinence, www.incontinence.org

Includes simple overviews of diagnostic and treatment options for incontinence, a message board, links to other helpful sites, and a physician referral network.

International Pelvic Pain Society (IPPS), www.pelvicpain.org

This organization is comprised of professionals engaged in pain management for women. The "Medical Links" section features many useful Web site resources.

Interstitial Cystitis Network, www.ic-network.com

The Interstitial Cystitis Network is dedicated to interstitial cystitis and other pelvic pain disorders. The site features a library where you can read the latest research abstracts and articles online, an archive of patient education materials on topics ranging from diagnostic techniques to treatments and self-care, an on-line support group, and an area to review lectures from IC professionals worldwide.

Med Help International (MHI), www.medhelp.org

Med Help International is dedicated to helping patients find the highest quality medical information in the world today, offering patients the tools to assist in informed treatment decisions.

National Institutes of Health (NIH), www.nih.gov

The federal focal point for biomedical research in the United States.

National Women's Health Resource Center (NWHRC), www.healthywomen.org

This Web site offers comprehensive information on women's health topics.

OBGYN.net, www.obgyn.net

Addressing health conditions and medical procedures for women, this site features separate on-line discussion forums for patients and medical professionals, plus an abundance of articles, links, and editorials.

Pelvicfloor.com, www.pelvicfloor.com

Sponsored by the author of this book, Dr. Magnus Murphy, the site contains valuable information on surgical techniques and an image and document library. Importantly, the site is a discussion forum for women worldwide, who log in to discuss a wide range of pelvic floor disorders. In many cases, Dr. Murphy personally answers posts.

Urology Channel, www.urologychannel.com

Board certified physicians develop and monitor the content of Urology Channel as a part of healthcommunities.com, a Web site designed to raise the quality of consumer health care information services. Find clearly explained, medically accurate information regarding urologic conditions; ask questions of a board-certified urologist; and view videos of common surgeries.

Urogynecologychannel.com, www.urogynecologychannel.com

This is the Web site for the Atlanta Center for Laparoscopic Urogynecology, a women's care facility dedicated exclusively to urogynecology, female incontinence, and reconstructive vaginal surgery. John R. Miklos M.D., FACOG, heads the practice located at 3400-C Old Milton Pkwy., Ste. 330, Alpharetta (Atlanta), GA 30005, 770-475-4499.

Women's Health, http://womenshealth.about.com/msub6.htm

Information about urinary incontinence, urinary tract infections, and other bladder conditions in women can be found here.

Women's Health Channel, www.womenshealthchannel.com

Visitors will find information regarding women's health conditions. They can ask questions of a women's health professional, view videos of common surgeries, and read patient and health care practitioner interviews.

Training

Biofeedback Certification Institute of America (BCIA), 10200 W. 44th Ave., Ste. 310, Wheat Ridge, CO 80033-2840, Web site: www.bcia.org, E-mail: bcia@resourcenter.com. The primary mission of BCIA is to protect the public welfare by assuring the competence of certified biofeedback practitioners. BCIA policies and procedures are determined by an independent board of directors, which is comprised of a rotating group of distinguished biofeedback clinicians, researchers, and educators.

Biofeedback Foundation of Europe (BFE), P.O. Box 75416, 1070 AK, Amsterdam, The Netherlands, 31 20 44 22 631, Web site: www.bfe.org, E-mail: mail@bfe.org. The Biofeedback Foundation of Europe (BFE) was founded to promote a greater awareness of biofeedback among European health professionals and, through training workshops, educate clinicians in the use of biofeedback techniques and technology.

Griffiths Urodynamics and Pro-Continence Consulting (GUPC), Room 3A05, Edmonton General Site, 11111 Jasper Ave., Edmonton, AB T5K 0L4, Canada, 780-482-8914, Web site: http://ourworld.compuserve.com/homepages/nacs, E-mail: nacs@compuserve.com. Professionals (R.N. and M.D.) and nonprofessionals (caregivers with little or no training) can get access to advice and training courses in incontinence assessment and management through this Web site.

Southern Biofeedback Corporation (SBC), 4271 Chatham Crest Ln., Sugar Hill, GA 30518, 800-227-5197 or 770-614-7239, Web site: www.southernbiofeedback.com, E-mail: Nschully@concentric.net. This site provides instrumentation and training for biofeedback applications.

Urodynamics training, 800-522-6743 or 802-878-1110, Web site: www.laborie.com, E-mail: kjankowski@laborie.com. Derek Griffiths teaches hands-on urodynamics courses under the auspices of Laborie Medical Technologies, with participation of a host urologist or specialist in incontinence. Interested visitors to the site can get information on the two-and-a-half-day courses at sites in North America, China, and Australia.

MISCELLANEOUS

Continence Restored, Inc. (CRI), 407 Strawberry Hill Ave., Stamford, CT 06902, 203-348-0601. Persons with incontinence and their families and friends can express concerns and receive assistance here. The organization also offers information on bladder control and phone assistance in starting support groups.

Agency for Health Care Policy and Research (AHCPR), U.S. Department of Health and Human Services, Public Health Service Publication Clearinghouse, P.O. Box 8547, Silver Spring, MD 20907, 800-358-9295, Web site: www.ahcprq.gov. This federal organization arranges for the development, review, and updating of clinical practice guidelines. The clinical practice guideline is produced in several versions, each created to meet the particular needs of its readers. The patient guide, written for patients and their families, describes the condition and treatment options in easy-to-understand terms. The booklet can help patients share in decisions about their own health care. Copies of the guidelines can be obtained at no charge by calling toll free.

The National Women's Health Information Center (NWHIC), 800-994-9662 or 800-994-WOMAN, Web site: www.4woman.gov. The National Women's Health Information Center (NWHIC) is a federal government source for women's health information. NWHIC's mission is to provide current, reliable, commercial, and cost-free health information to women and their families.

Society for Women's Health Research (SWHR), 1828 L St., N.W., Ste. 625, Washington, DC 20036, 202-223-8224, Web site: www.womens-health.org, E-mail: info@womens-health.org. The Society for Women's Health Research is the United States's only not-for-profit organization whose sole mission is to improve the health of women through research. The Society advocates increased funding for research on women's health; encourages the study of sex differences that may affect the prevention, diagnosis, and treatment of disease; and promotes the inclusion of women in medical research studies.

APPENDIX B
History of Cesarean Section

The origin of the word "cesarean," or caesarian (British spelling), is unclear. The word is rumored to have originated from Julius Caesar, who it is believed, was the first live infant born by this method (in 100 B.C.E.). This is very doubtful, especially in light of the fact that his mother, Aurelia, survived his birth, and that written history contains no record of such an event. In fact, Aurelia was still alive when Caesar was forty-eight years old. Her survival is almost certainly incompatible with a cesarean birth, since the maternal mortality (death rate) after cesarean was almost 100 percent until the early part of this century.

It is almost impossible for the modern reader to understand the fear, horror, and revulsion that the concept of cesarean birth engendered until relatively recently. To try and understand the history of this operation previously known as the delivery of a child "per viam non naturalem" (by non-natural route), one has to understand something about the surgical practices of previous times. Until the early 1900s, the procedure was usually performed without any anesthetic whatsoever. Four or five men would hold the woman down on a table (often a kitchen table), while the surgeon would cut into her abdomen with a dirty kitchen knife or pocketknife, or sometimes a razor blade. This knife or blade was often caked with old blood and grime, while the surgeon's hands were often even dirtier.

Surgeons would walk from patient to patient, and even from corpses to patients, without washing their hands. Their status was, to some degree, dependent on the built-up gore and blood on their coats. The most important criterion distinguishing a good surgeon from a bad one was the speed at which the particular operation could be performed. The lack of effective and safe anesthetics makes this understandable and logical, but it doesn't lend itself to the development of safe and anatomically correct surgical practices.

The surgeon would cut through the abdominal wall and through the uterus, pull the baby out, and then sew the *skin* incision but leave the underlying tissues, including the uterine incision, open. Women almost invariably bled to death, and those few who survived this stage of the operation, almost certainly succumbed later to overwhelming infection. Remember that antibiotics only date from the 1930s.

As a result of the exceedingly poor maternal outcome, the procedure was usually only performed after the death of the mother or when she was definitely at death's door.

In the Roman Empire the division of the so-called Justinian Corpus Juris contained the "Rex Regia" law. This law, enacted by the second king of Rome, Numa Pompilius (715–673 B.C.E.), stated that it was forbidden to bury a dead pregnant woman before the fetus has been removed. This was also the practice in India, Arabia, Persia, and possibly even in early Egypt.

In 1609, Jacques Guillemeau, writing of the "happy deliverie of women," notes: "*Lawiers judge them worthy of death, who shall burie a great bellyed-woman that is dead, before the child be taken foorth.*" He then goes on to speak of the haste needed to save the baby, but also about the need to ensure that the woman is dead and that "*her kinsfolkes, friends and others that are present, do all affirme and confesse, that her Soule is departed.*"[1] He himself had twice performed cesarean sections on living mothers, and had seen several more done by three Paris surgeons. All the women died. Nevertheless there are some occasional reports of women surviving their ordeals and even going on to deliver babies vaginally later. In the eighteenth century, thirty-six living infants were reported to have been delivered by cesarean after their mother's death, and by the mid-nineteenth century, over eighty more such cases had been reported. Before 1700, assessments are difficult since the Lazarus-like accounts of living babies rescued from their dead mother's womb, some buried for days, strain the credibility of even the most gullible.

Even Shakespeare took note of this interesting operation in *Macbeth,* when he writes: "*Macduff was from his mother's womb untimely ripped.*"

The earliest account of this procedure in any medical textbook of importance appeared about the year 1350, where it is noted to be a proper procedure after the death of the mother. The oldest authentic record of a living child born by cesarean, however, is that of Gorgias, the celebrated orator of Sicily in 508 B.C.E. Another early cesarean survivor was Scipio Africanus (born in 237 B.C.E., and also called "Caesar"), the conqueror of Hannibal.

Greek mythology contains some references to such an unnatural birth. Asclepios, the tutelary god of medicine, was delivered from his mother, Coronis, in this manner: "*Natum flammis uteroque parentis eripuit geminique tulit Chironis in antrum.*" (He snatched his son from his mother's womb, says Ovid, saved him from the flames, and carried him to the cave of the centaur, Chiron). Hermes was the alleged surgeon after her husband Apollo's sister, Artemis, had killed Coronis.

Although this operation is mentioned in the Talmud and in the Veda books of India, some noted physicians of antiquity do not even mention it in their works. Aulus Aurelius Cornelius Celsus does not mention the operation in books vii and viii of his *De Medicina* which deal with surgical treatment. Similarly, Soranus of Ephesus, regarded as the greatest obstetrician and gynecologist of antiquity, who lived from 98 to 138 C.E., and whose published works commanded the utmost respect for 1500 years, did not mention the cesarean method of delivery. Other important obstetricians, among them Aetius of Amida and Paulus Aegineta, who both published important obstetrical works, were silent on the topic. That such eminent physicians of the time ignored the operation suggests that it was an extremely rare occurrence and that it was not part of practical obstetrics. It may also be that the medical politics of the time, or disdain for the almost uniformly poor outcome of the surgery, led to a conscious choice to exclude the topic. As mentioned, the origin of the word "caesarian" is very uncertain and it is unlikely that there will ever be a unanimous opinion. I already mentioned that Julius Caesar was unlikely to have been born by "caesarian." Furthermore, the word predates him by centuries, since Scipio Africanus was also named "Caesar" and Pliny's *Natural History* records a Caesar before the Samnite wars in about 340 B.C.E. Gaius Pliny the Elder was the first to use the term "Caesonis," indicating "one cut from his mother's womb" and, in this respect, Scipio Africanus could be said to be the first Caesar.

The derivation of the term remains unclear, however, and several far-fetched theories have been suggested. These range from "caesa," which means "elephant," in the Moorish and Punic languages (Julius Caesar was a large man), to "caesaries" (a bushy head of hair), to "caesius" (to have blue-gray eyes). In Roman use, the term "Caedere" indicated killing, slaying, or destroying on a grand scale (which could easily be understood to be associated with the "Caesar"), whereas "secare" or "incidere" meant to cut or incise. After the murder of Julius Caesar (definitely a "caedes"), his assassins took on the name Caesar, thus belying any supposed connection between the name and any specific manner of birth quite convincingly.

Further analysis of the word "caesarian" reveals other interesting meanings. "Caesarianus" means belonging to Caesar, whereas "caesariatus" means longhaired. "Caesareus" also depicts an ownership of, or being part of Caesar.

It was the Jesuit, Théophile Raynaud, who first used the term "caesareus" in the title of his book, which was the first to be written on the "caesarean" operation. François Rousset gave the first verifiable account of a successful cesarean section, which resulted in the survival not only of the child, but also of the mother, sometime in the 1500s, although he called the operation a "hysterotomotokie." This term is more in line with current use of the term "hysterotomy," which is a similar operation to a cesarean but done for a nonviable fetus, or *any* incision into the uterine cavity, even in the nonpregnant woman. Anyway, this "hysterotomotokie" was performed by none other than a sow gelder, named Jacob Nufer of Siegertshaufen, which is about twelve and a half miles southwest of Augsburg, Germany. He did this around 1500 C.E. on his own wife, and used a razor blade. Apparently, she had been in labor for many days, and over a dozen midwives and barbers had failed to deliver the baby. Even though his wife was in favor of the attempt, since she believed that she was dying anyway, the authorities turned deaf ears to his petitions. Nufer, in desperation, proceeded anyway. After laying her on a table with the necessary attendants to hold her down, Nufer made the incision, extracted the child and apparently sutured the abdominal wall. Almost miraculously his wife recovered, and just as remarkably went on to bear twins at a later date and four more children, all of whom were delivered vaginally.

Although the operation was repeated intermittently throughout the following centuries in different countries, it was always done as a last resort on a living mother. As a result of the extremely high maternal mortality, most eminent obstetricians not only frowned on the procedure but also openly condemned it, so no progress or uniformity of technique was achieved. There was even an active anti-cesarean movement, called "École anti-Cesarienne" led by Jean-François Sacombe in postrevolution France.

As is common with most human endeavors, jealousy and rivalry enter into the history of this remarkable operation. Although it is widely believed that Jessee Bennett of Mason County, West Virginia, performed the second wholly successful cesarean in the world and the first in the New World in 1794 (again, on his own wife), this same honor is also claimed for John Lambert Richmond (near Cincinnati, Ohio) in 1827. Other claims place this second event in Martinique in 1805.

The accounts and assessments of Bennett's operation contain allegations of fraud, intrigue, and all the necessary ingredients for a good story. For one thing, it is alleged he graduated from the University of Pennsylvania, but apparently there are no records of any such graduation. The accounts of the operation and of Bennett's life supposedly hinge on the article by A. L. Knight entitled "The Life and Times of Jessee Bennett, M.D." This was published fifty years after Bennett's death and the only source of information was apparently what either Bennett or his sister-in-law, Nancy Hawkins, had told Knight at least fifty-three years earlier. This would have made A. L. Knight between fourteen and eighteen years old!

Each individual country has divergent histories about the progress of the operation before this century. So, for instance, in Great Britain, a surgeon James Barlow of Lancashire performed the first operation of this kind where the life of the mother was saved, while he worked in Chorley in 1793. In Sweden, the first recorded cesarean section was performed in 1360 C.E. This section was performed postmortem, after the death of the mother. During the years 1758–1875, thirteen cesarean sections were performed in Sweden. All of the women died. During 1882–1890, thirteen more cesarean sections were performed using a new method and with the loss of about 54 percent of the women. The first cesarean on a living woman in Australia was performed in 1872, and, in South Africa, sometime between 1815 and 1821. The South African child, James Barry Munnik, survived, and his grandson, James Barry Munnik Hertzog (1866–1942), later became the prime minister of South Africa from 1924 to 1939.

During the subsequent decades, tremendous medical advances were made in the fields of microbiology, which led to increasingly effective antiseptic technique, surgical technique, and anesthetics. As the figures for maternal mortality after cesarean section plummeted, the procedure became more accepted and established.

NOTE

1. Jacques Guillemeau, *De l'hereux accouchement des femmes* (Happy Delivery of Women) (Paris: Nicolas Buon, 1609).

Glossary

Altriciality: Relative underdevelopment of the human newborn infant compared to other primates. Resultant from shortened gestation.

Anal sphincters: The muscles in the anus (opening to the rectum).

Anesthesia: Loss of sensation in any part of the body induced by a numbing or paralyzing agent. Often used during surgery to put a person to sleep.

Antepartum: The predelivery pregnant period.

Anterior: Top or upper.

Antibacterial: Type of medication used to kill bacteria that cause infection.

Anticholinergic: A drug that interferes with the effects of acetylcholine. These drugs assist with bladder storage by decreasing bladder contractions and are used to treat urge incontinence.

Anti-incontinence surgery: The use of surgical procedures to treat urinary incontinence (see also *artificial urinary sphincter, bladder suspension, periurethral bulking injections, sling procedures*).

Anus: The final two inches of the rectum, surrounded by the internal anal sphincter and the external sphincter. Stool is passed through the anus, which is an opening or aperture.

Artificial urinary sphincter: A mechanical device surgically implanted into the patient that consists of a cuff placed around the bulbar urethra or bladder neck, a pressure-regulating balloon, and a pump. The device is used to control opening and closing of the urethra manually and is the most commonly used surgical procedure for the treatment of male urethral insufficiency.

Atonic bladder: Also referred to as a lower motor neuron bladder. Often caused by peripheral neuropathies, such as diabetes mellitus. The bladder is flaccid and overdistended with urine and overflow incontinence may occur.

Atrophy: Thinning and decreased blood flow to tissue resulting from a lack of hormones, most commonly estrogen.

Behavioral techniques: Specific treatments designed to alter the relationship between the patient's symptoms and his/her behavior and/or environment for the treatment of maladaptive urinary voiding patterns. This may be achieved by modification of the behavior and/or environment of the patient (see also *biofeedback therapy, bladder training, electrical stimulation, habit training, pelvic muscle exercises, prompted voiding*).

Biofeedback therapy: A behavioral technique in which a person learns how to consciously control involuntary responses such as muscle contractions. The person receives a visual, auditory, or tactile signal (the feedback) that indicates how well the person's muscles are responding to the commands of the education process to accomplish a specific therapeutic result. The signal is displayed in a quantitative way, and the patient is taught how to alter it and thus control the physiologic process. This technique is used most often to teach pelvic muscle exercises.

Bipedal: Walking erect on two legs.

Bladder: The bladder is a muscular organ, which lies in the pelvis and is supported by the pelvic floor muscles. The bladder has only two functions: to stretch to allow the storage of urine and to contract to enable the expulsion of urine. The term "detrusor" is used to refer to the smooth muscle structure of the bladder.

Bladder capacity: The amount (maximum volume) of urine that the bladder can hold. Often referred to as bladder volume.

Bladder diary or record: A daily record of bladder habits, documenting voiding (urination) and episodes of incontinence.

Bladder neck: Junction between urethra and bladder.

Bladder suspension: Also called bladder neck suspension. A term for several surgical procedures employed to treat urethral hypermobility by elevating and securing the bladder to its proper position within the body. Used for stress UI.

Bladder training: A behavioral technique that requires the person to resist or inhibit the sensation of urgency (the strong desire to urinate), to postpone voiding, and to urinate according to a timetable rather than to the urge to void.

Bladder ultrasound or bladder scan: A method of measuring the urine that remains in the bladder. This is a test that is used to diagnose incomplete bladder emptying. An ultrasound uses sound waves to measure the urine volume. It is painless and does not involve the use of radiation like X rays.

Bone anchors: A type of surgery for stress UI that uses "bone anchors" by drilling screws into the pelvic (pubic) bone to secure and lift (suspend) the bladder in a fixed position.

Bowel movement: The act of passing feces (stool) through the anus.

Bowels: Another word for intestines or colon.

Catheter: A narrow flexible tube that is inserted into the urethra and into the bladder for the purpose of draining urine or performing diagnostic tests of bladder or urethral function.

Catheterization: A procedure in which a catheter is passed through the urethra and into the bladder for the purpose of draining urine and performing diagnostic tests of bladder or urethral function.

Cerebral cortex: The part of the brain that is the master control center for voluntary (conscious) control of voiding (urination). Often referred to as the "bladder micturition center," the cerebral cortex commands the bladder to hold urine until a socially acceptable time when voiding can occur.

Cervix: The tip of the uterus; also the intravaginal part of the uterus. This needs to open before delivery can occur. This is where Pap smears are taken from.

Cholinergic: Fibers in the parasympathetic nervous system that release a chemical called acetylcholine.

Classical cesarean section: Cesarean section where the incision in the uterine muscle is made through the thickest part of the uterus, vertically. This leads to future significantly increased risk for rupture of the scar.

Compliance: A term used for the bladder to determine its ability to stretch or expand. Persons can have a "poorly compliant bladder," which means that the bladder does not stretch as well and holds smaller amounts of urine (small capacity).

Constipation: A condition in which bowel movements are infrequent, hard, and dry, and elimination of feces is difficult and infrequent.

Continence: The ability to exercise voluntary control over the urge (intense sensation to go), to void (urinate), or defecate until an appropriate time and place can be found to void (or have a bowel movement).

Cystitis: Irritation or inflammation (swelling) of the bladder usually caused by an infection.

Cystocele: Prolapse of the bladder into the vagina. This can be seen as a bulge from the anterior wall of the vagina.

Cystometry (cystometrogram): A test used to assess the function of the bladder by measuring the pressure/volume as the bladder is slowly being filled. Cystometry is used to assess bladder urge sensation, capacity, and compliance. There are different variations of the test depending on the problem being investigated, but regardless of the technique, cystometry involves insertion of a catheter into the bladder.

Cystourethrography: The use of X-ray imaging to examine the urinary bladder and urethra. In voiding cystourethrography, an X-ray picture of the bladder and urethra is obtained during urination.

Cystoscopy: Also sometimes called cystourethroscopy. A procedure used to diagnose urinary tract disorders and provide a direct view of the urethra and bladder by inserting a flexible scope into the urethra and then into the bladder.

Decreased bladder compliance: A failure to store urine in the bladder, caused by the loss of bladder wall elasticity and of bladder accommodation. This condition may result from radiation cystitis or from inflammatory bladder conditions such as chemical cystitis, interstitial cystitis, and certain neurologic bladder disorders.

Defecate: The act of having a bowel movement.

Dehydration: A state that occurs when not enough fluid is present to fulfill the body's fluid needs.

Dementia: General loss of short- and long-term memory and mental deterioration. It may affect emotions, abstract thinking, judgment, impulse control, and learning and can cause functional incontinence.

Denervation: Loss of neuronal connections.

Detrusor: In the urinary system, the detrusor muscle is the smooth muscle in the wall of the bladder that contracts the bladder and expels the urine. The bladder is often referred to as the detrusor muscle.

Detrusor hyperactivity with impaired bladder contractility (DHIC): A condition characterized by involuntary detrusor contractions in which patients either are unable to empty their bladder completely or can empty their bladder completely only with straining due to poor contractility of the detrusor.

Detrusor hyperreflexia or instability (unstable or spastic bladder): Involuntary and irregular detrusor contraction in the presence of associated neurologic disorders, often causes urge incontinence-like symptoms.

Detrusor instability: Instability of the bladder muscle leading to uninhibited, abnormal bladder contractions. This leads to urgency or urgency incontinence.

Detrusor sphincter dyssynergia (DSD): An inappropriate contraction of the external sphincter concurrent with an involuntary contraction of the detrusor. In the adult, DSD is a common feature of neurologic voiding disorders.

Devascularization: Loss of vascular connections.

Dilatation: To dilate; to stretch, as in "dilatation of the urethra" or "dilatation and curretage" (D&C).

Disimpaction: The act of removing stool from the rectum, which could not be eliminated normally. Enemas, suppositories, laxatives, and finger extraction are all means of disimpacting stool.

Dysuria: Painful or difficult urination, most frequently caused by infection or inflammation, but certain drugs can also cause it.

Ehlers-Danlos syndrome: A genetically determined and inherited disorder of collagen tissues (the body's connective tissue). Patients with this disorder have increased risks of joint injuries, hernias (including pelvic hernias), as well as blood vessel complications like aneurisms.

Elective cesarean birth: Delivery of baby by planned cesarean section.

Electrical stimulation: A treatment that is an application of an electric current to the pelvic floor muscles and bladder to cause a muscle contraction. This treatment is used in patients who have nerve damage to the bladder or pelvis. It may also be used to help identify the muscle. This is characterized as a behavioral treatment.

Electromyography (EMG): A diagnostic test that is used to measure the electrical activity of the muscles, bladder, and the pelvic floor muscles.

Endopelvic fascia: The fascia of the inner pelvis.

Enterocele: A true herniation into the top of the vagina. This results from loops of small bowel herniating through a fascia tear into the space between the pelvic fascia and the vaginal wall.

Enuresis: The involuntary loss of urine (urinary incontinence) during sleep. This term is most often applied to bedwetting in children.

Episiotomy: An incision made in the lower vulva, to increase the vaginal outlet aperture.

Estrogen: A hormone in women produced primarily by the ovaries. Estrogen is believed to play a major role in maintaining the strength and tone of the urethra and the pelvic floor.

Evacuation: Another word for a bowel movement.

External sphincter: The outer layer of the sphincter, usually under voluntary control.

Fascia: Connective tissue supporting organ structures. Consisting of mostly collagen fibers, this tissue makes up ligaments, keeps muscular bundles together, and lends structural integrity and strength to the body.

Fecal incontinence: The accidental and involuntary loss of liquid or solid stool or gas from the anus.

Fecal impaction: A mass of stool (feces) that remains packed in the rectum rather than being passed normally. Impaction can contribute to incontinence by irritating the urethra; causing urge UI; or by blocking the urethra, preventing the bladder from emptying, and completely causing overflow incontinence.

Feces (stool): Waste material produced from the intestines. Feces are composed of bacteria, undigested food, and material produced from the intestines.

Fecundity: Number of children.

Fetus: The intrauterine unborn infant.

Fistula: An opening between two organs (between the bladder and vagina in women or the bladder and the rectum in men). Women with a fistula may have urinary incontinence.

Flatus: Bowel gas.

Flatulence: The release of gas through the anus.

Forceps delivery: Delivery accomplished by the obstetrical forceps.

Frequency: An abnormally frequent desire to void usually more than eight times a day, often of only small amounts (e.g., less than 7 fluid ounces [200 ml]).

Gas: Material that results from swallowed air, air produced from certain foods, or that is created when bacteria in the colon break down waste material. Gas that is released from the rectum is called flatulence.

Genuine stress urinary incontinence: Incontinence related to episodes of increased intra-abdominal pressure.

Gestation: Length of pregnancy.

Gynecologist: Physician specializing in female disorders, particularly those of the reproductive and urological organs.

Habit training: A behavioral technique that calls for scheduled toileting at regular intervals to prevent incontinence. Unlike bladder training, there is no systematic effort to motivate the person to delay voiding and resist urge.

Hematoma: Blood clot.

Hematuria: Blood in the urine.

Hypermobility: A term that is applied to the urethra. When the urethra becomes hypermobile it will drop from its normal position during physical activity and may result in stress UI.

Hysterectomy: Surgical removal of the uterus.

Idiopathic: Applied to a medical problem or disease when the cause is unknown.

Impaction: A blockage of stool in the rectum, usually composed of a large amount of dried stool that is difficult to evacuate.

Incidence: New occurrences of a disorder per year.

Incontinence: Loss of normal bodily control over the storage role of a particular organ.

Incontinence, anal/fecal incontinence: Loss of storage mechanism of rectum. This means loss of control over flatus or stool.

Incontinence, urinary incontinence: Loss of control over urinary storage function, thus leakage of urine.

Induction of labor: The process of initiating and expediting labor and delivery.

Informed consent: A contractual agreement between a patient and a physician, whereby the patient gives permission to undergo a certain procedure based on as clear an understanding of the issues as is possible. This understanding should be based on education and explanation.

Innervation: Connection with intact nerves. This is used in conjunction with muscles.

Intermittency: Interruption of the urinary stream while voiding.

Intermittent catheterization: The use of catheters inserted through the urethra into the bladder every three to six hours for bladder drainage in persons with urinary retention.

Internal sphincter: The internal layer of the sphincter, usually under involuntary control.

Intra-abdominal: Inside the abdominal cavity.

Intrauterine: Inside the uterus.

Intravesical pressure: Refers to the pressure within the bladder.

Intrinsic sphincter deficiency: A weakening of the muscles around the bladder neck.

Invasive: As in "invasive procedures." Procedures involving interference to change an outcome. It could also mean penetrating, or entering, the temporal order of the proceedings, or the physical body.

Involuntary detrusor (bladder) contraction: A bladder contraction that is not under voluntary control. This can cause urge urinary incontinence, detrusor hyperreflexia, detrusor instability, and spastic bladder.

Kegel exercises: Contraction of the pelvic floor muscles that support the bladder, uterus, and rectum. These exercises were developed in the 1940s by obstetrician and gynecologist Dr. Arnold Kegel.

Kidneys: Organs that continually filter the blood to separate out waste products, which are combined with excess water to form urine.

Laparoscopic surgery: Surgery using a laparoscope and minimal-access incisions. In this way, large skin incisions are avoided.

Late complications: Complications that occur significantly later than the causal event.

Levator ani: The main muscle of the pelvic floor made up of different parts. These parts include pubococcygeus, iliococcygeus, coccygeus, and ischeococcygeus.

Marfan syndrome: A genetically determined and inherited disorder of collagen tissues (the body's connective tissue). Patients with this disorder have increased risks of joint injuries, hernias (including pelvic hernias), and blood vessel complications like aneurisms.

Meatus: The opening to the urethra.

Mesh: Like a net, web, or screen. A mesh material may be used to support the bladder in certain surgery for stress UI.

Micturition: Another term for urination or voiding.

Midwife: Nonphysician practitioner attending and helping during labor and delivery. Midwives are often, but not always, nurses.

Mixed urinary incontinence: The combination, in a patient, of urge urinary incontinence and stress urinary incontinence (see *urgency incontinence, stress urinary incontinence*).

Morbidity: The development of complications.

Mortality: Death.

Mucosa: Epithelial tissue encountered in the mouth, vagina, anus, etc.

Natural childbirth: A term normally used to indicate the natural order of childbirth as in the "natural" state. In reality, this would mean total noninterference by attendants. The term is used loosely, meaning different things by different people.

Neonatology: The specialty of looking after newborn babies.

Nervous system: The nervous system is made up of nerves that are voluntary and involuntary and is composed of the brain, the spinal cord, and the sensory nerves. The nervous system carries messages to the brain from the body and motor nerves, which provide messages from the brain to the muscles and which help muscles function.

Neurogenic bladder: An atonic or unstable bladder associated with a neurological disease condition, such as diabetes, stroke, or spinal cord injury.

Nocturia: Awakening at night by the need to void. As a person ages, the number of times he or she awakens to void will increase.

Nocturnal enuresis: The involuntary loss of urine (urinary incontinence) in adults that occurs during sleep. This term is most often used for bedwetting in children.

Overactive bladder: A condition characterized by involuntary detrusor (bladder) contractions during the time the bladder is filling, which may be spontaneous or provoked and which the patient cannot suppress. Symptoms include urinary urgency, frequency, and nocturia and may include urge incontinence.

Overflow incontinence: The involuntary loss of urine associated with overdistension of the bladder. Overflow incontinence results from urinary retention that causes the capacity of the bladder to be overwhelmed. Continuous or intermittent leakage of a small amount of urine results.

Parasympathetic: A part of the autonomic nervous system. Parasympathetic (cholinergic) activity causes contraction of the bladder and assists in the voiding process. Emptying of the bladder is primarily a parasympathetic activity.

Parity: Number of babies at gestational term.

Pelvic floor: The floor of the abdominal cavity. It pertains to those structures that form the natural bottom of the pelvic and intra-abdominal cavities.

Pelvic floor dysfunction: Disorders of the pelvic floor related to physiological or anatomical abnormalities. They include incontinence, prolapse, pain syndromes, and others.

Pelvic floor muscles: The hammock or sling of muscles in the pelvic floor that normally assists in maintaining continence by supporting the pelvic organs (bladder, uterus, and rectum).

Pelvic muscle exercises (PMEs): A treatment that requires repetitive active exercise of the pubococcygeus muscle. Exercising these muscles will improve urethral resistance and urinary control by strengthening the periurethral and pelvic muscles. Also called Kegel exercises or pelvic floor exercises.

Pelvic nerve plexus: A nerve plexus is a collection of nerves that are bundled together and contain many nerves coming from different organs or parts of the same organ, or from different spinal roots. Nerve plexuses also contain many different types of nerves, such as sensory nerves (afferent, ascending or taking messages toward the spine or brain), and motor nerves (efferent, descending or taking messages toward the target organ).

Pelvis: The ring of bones at the lower end of the trunk within which the pelvic organs lie.

Percutaneous: To place or perform a procedure underneath the skin. No incision (cutting) is necessary.

Perinatal: Viable fetus prebirth, up to seven days after birth.

Perineal body: The thickened part between the anal and vaginal openings.

Perineometer: An instrument originally invented by Dr. Arnold Kegel to measure the strength of the pelvic muscle contractions. An electronic perineometer is used in electronyogram (EMG) biofeedback training.

Perineum: Area between the anus and vagina in women, and anus and base of scrotum and penis in men.

Peritoneum: Thin shiny layer of tissue covering the inner wall of the abdominal cavity.

Periurethral bulking injections: A surgical treatment for urethral sphincter deficiency that involves injecting materials such as polytetrafluoroethylene (PTFE) or collagen into the periurethral area to increase urethral compression.

Pessary: A silicone device that is placed in the vagina to provide support.

Pharmacological treatment: The use of medications to treat urinary incontinence.

Placenta accreta: Stuck placenta resulting from placental tissue growing into the uterine wall.

Placenta previa: Blocking placenta. The placenta lies over the internal cervix, covering the passage the baby needs to take to be born.

Polyuria: Excretion of a large volume of urine during a certain interval of time. It can be a result of uncontrolled diabetes mellitus or after taking a diuretic.

Postvoid residual (PVR) volume: The amount of fluid remaining in the bladder immediately following the completion of voiding. A PVR can be estimated by abdominal palpation (feeling the stomach) and percussion or bimanual examination. Specific measurement of PVR volume can be accomplished by catheterization, pelvic ultrasound, radiography, or radioisotope studies.

Posterior: Bottom or lower.

Postpartum: After delivery. This period lasts until six weeks after delivery.

Prevalence: Occurrence of a disorder in the general population.

Prognosis: Prediction of most likely future outcome.

Prolapse: Falling out of, falling down, dropping, or bulging.

Prompted voiding: A behavioral technique for primarily dependent or cognitively impaired persons. Prompted voiding in the incontinent person attempts to teach awareness of incontinence status and to request toileting assistance, either independently or after being prompted by a caregiver.

Pubic symphysis: Pubic (pelvic) bone that lies under the mons pubis.

Pubococcygeus muscle: Another name for the levator ani muscle, one of the pelvic muscles that hold the pelvic organ in place.

Pudendal nerve: Main nerve supplying the pelvic floor, bladder, and urethra. Damage to this nerve can cause incontinence.

Rectocele: Prolapse of the rectum into the vagina. This can be seen as a bulge from the lower wall of the vagina.

Rectovaginal septum: The fascial layer that separates the vagina from the rectum.

Rectum: Last segment of colon, or large intestine; the lowest part of the bowel found right before the anus.

Rectus muscle: Longitudinal abdominal muscles. These are the midline muscles leading to the well-recognized dimpling in well-built bodybuilders.

Rectus sheath: The fascial sheath surrounding the rectus muscles.

Retention: Inability to empty urine from the bladder, which can be caused by atonic bladder or obstruction of the urethra.

Risk factor: Quality that makes a person more susceptible to a specific disease.

Sacrospinous ligament: Ligament attaching the ischial spine to the sacrum.

Second stage: That stage of labor where the cervix has fully opened up.

Sensory urgency: Urgency associated with bladder hypersensitivity (see *urge, urgency*).

Sling procedures: Surgical methods for treating urinary incontinence involving the placement of a sling under the urethrovesical junction and anchored to abdominal structures. The sling is made either from tissue obtained from the person undergoing the sling procedure or from tissue obtained from another source (e.g., mesh).

Sphincter: Circular muscle which closes off a hollow organ during contraction.

Spinal anesthetic: The anesthetic solution is injected into the spinal canal immediately surrounding the spinal column. No catheter is used and the needle used is thus thinner. Spinals cannot be "topped up."

Spinal fluid: Fluid surrounding the spinal column and brain.

Stress urinary incontinence: A form of urinary incontinence characterized by the involuntary loss of urine from the urethra during physical exertion; for example, during coughing. The stress incontinence symptom or complaint may be confirmed by observing urine loss at the same time that there is an increase in abdominal pressure (e.g., during coughing, laughing). Urine leakage occurs in the absence of a detrusor (bladder) contraction or an overdistended bladder (see *hypermobility* of bladder neck and *intrinsic sphincter deficiency*).

Stress maneuvers: Activities that increase pressure in the bladder, such as coughing and laughing; this is a diagnostic test to check for stress UI.

Suprapubic: Above the pubic bone.

Suprapubic cystostomy: A surgical procedure involving insertion of a tube or similar instrument through the anterior abdominal (stomach) wall above the symphysis pubis into the bladder to permit urine drainage from the bladder.

Sympathetic nervous system: A part of the nervous system that causes relaxation of the bladder and contraction of the internal sphincter. Urine storage in the bladder is primarily the result of a functional sympathetic system.

Thromboembolisis: Blood clotting and migration of clots to plug distant blood vessels.

Transient urinary incontinence: Temporary episodes of urinary incontinence that are reversible once the cause or causes of the episode(s) are identified and treated.

Trigone: The most sensitive area on the inside (wall) of the bladder, where bladder nerves are most highly concentrated.

Ultrasonography: A technique that uses ultrasound to obtain visual images of the urinary tract for the purpose of assessing its anatomic status.

Underactive bladder: A condition characterized by a bladder contraction of inadequate magnitude and/or duration to effect bladder emptying in a normal time span. Drugs, fecal impaction, and neurologic conditions such as diabetic neuropathy or low spinal cord injury or as a result of radical pelvic surgery can cause this condition. It also can result from a weakening of the detrusor muscle from vitamin B_{12} deficiency or idiopathic causes. Bladder underactivity may cause overdistension of the bladder, resulting in overflow incontinence (see *overflow incontinence*).

Ureter: The muscular tubes carrying urine from kidneys to bladder.

Urethra: The tubular structure carrying urine from the bladder to the outside.

Urethral dilatation: A procedure in which a metal rod, called a dilator, is passed through the urethra for the purpose of stretching the urethra or opening a urethral stricture.

Urethral obstruction: Blockage of the urethra causing difficulty with urination, usually caused by a stricture or, in men, by an enlarged prostate.

Urethral stricture: Narrowing of the urethra.

Urethral pressure profilometry (UPP): A technique used to measure resting and dynamic pressures in the urethra.

Urethral sphincter mechanism: The segment of the urethra that influences storage and emptying of urine in the bladder. The urethral sphincter is like a "valve" that controls bladder emptying and voiding by tightening to close off the flow of urine or by relaxing, which opens the outlet from the bladder, allowing urine to flow from the bladder to the outside of the body. A deficiency of the urethral sphincter mechanism may allow leakage of urine in the absence of a detrusor (bladder) contraction.

Urethrocele: A hernia or dropping of the urethra allowing part of the urethra to press on the vaginal wall.

Urethrovesical: Connection or junction between the base of bladder (bladder neck) and urethra.

Urethrovesical angle: Angle formed by the base of the bladder and the urethra. Normal angle in women is 90 to 100 degrees. An increase in this angle causes stress UI. Bladder suspension surgery will correct the angle.

Urge: The sensation from the bladder producing the desire to void.

Urgency: A strong, intense desire to void immediately. It often accompanies frequency.

Urgency incontinence: Urinary incontinence related to involuntary bladder muscle contractions and an inability to suppress those contractions.

Urinary incontinence (UI): Involuntary or accidental loss of urine sufficient to be a problem. There are several types of UI, but all are characterized by an inability to restrain or control urinary voiding (see *mixed urinary incontinence, nocturnal enuresis, overflow incontinence, stress urinary incontinence, transient urinary incontinence, urgency incontinence*).

Urinary obstruction: Inability to void.

Urinary tract: Passageway from the pelvis of the kidney to the urinary orifice through the ureters, bladder, and urethra. There is an upper urinary tract (two kidneys and two ureters) and a lower urinary tract (bladder, sphincters, and urethra).

Urinary tract infection (UTI): An infection in the urinary tract caused by the invasion of disease-causing micro-organisms, which proceed to establish themselves, multiply, and produce various symptoms in their host. Infection of the bladder, better known as cystitis, is particularly common in women, mainly because of the much shorter urethra, which provides less of a barrier to bacteria.

Urodynamic assessment: Dynamic testing of the urological system whereby pressure differentials are measured.

Urodynamic tests: Tests designed to duplicate as nearly as possible the symptoms of incontinence in the way that you actually experience them. These tests determine the anatomic and functional status of the urinary bladder and urethra (see *cystometry, electromyography, urethral pressure profilometry, uroflowmetry, videourodynamics*).

Uroflowmetry: A urodynamic test that measures urine flow either visually, electronically, or with the use of a disposable flowmeter unit.

Urogenital: The structure pertaining to the urological and genital systems. Usually used when discussing the urogenital opening (opening at the bottom of the pelvic cavity through which the aforementioned organ systems run); or the urogenital diaphragm (simplistically seen as that part of the pelvic floor that supports the distal (farthest) ends of the urological system—the bladder neck and urethra—as well as the distal ends of the genitals, basically the vagina.

Uterine prolapse: The uterus has slipped (dropped) from its normal position and the cervix is closer to or may protrude outside the vagina.

Uterus: The womb.

Vacuum extraction: Delivery accomplished by the obstetrical vacuum.

Vagina: Also known as the birth canal. The vagina is a collapsible tube of smooth muscle with its opening located between the urethral orifice and the anal sphincter of women.

Vaginismus: Painful spasm of pelvic floor muscles in vaginal entry, such as during sexual intercourse.

Valsalva maneuver: The action of closing the airways and straining down on the abdominal muscles (such as when straining to have a bowel movement).

VBAC: Vaginal birth after previous cesarean.

Videourodynamics: A technique that combines the various urodynamic tests with simultaneous fluoroscopy. Fluoroscopy is a technique for examining internal structures by viewing the shadows cast on a fluorescent screen by objects or parts through which X rays are directed.

Voiding or bladder diary (record): Also called an "incontinence chart." A record maintained by the patient or caregiver that is used to record the frequency, timing, amount of voiding, and/or other factors associated with the patient's urinary incontinence.

Voiding reflex: The reflex in which the bladder indicates to the spinal cord that it is full of urine and the spinal cord then signals the bladder to contract and empty.

Voluntary control: Conscious control.

Vulvodynia: Painful vulva, also sometimes associated with urinary symptoms, painful intercourse, and generalized pelvic pain.

Selected References

Barrett, G., and C. R. Victor. "Incidence of Postnatal Dyspareunia." *British Journal of Sexual Medicine* 23, no. 5 (1996): 6–8.

Bergmans, L. C. M., H. J. M. Hendriks, K. Bo, et al. "Conservative Treatment of Stress Urinary Incontinence in Women." *British Journal of Urology* 82 (1998): 181–91.

Benson, J. T. *Female Pelvic Floor Disorders, Investigation and Management*. New York: W. W. Norton, 1992.

Blair Bell Research Society. Papers presented at the Royal College of Obstetricians and Gynaecologists, London, December 1997.

———. "Changes in the Urethral Sphincter in Relation to Child Birth and the Development." *British Journal of Obstetrics and Gynaecology* 105 (November 1998): 1220.

Brown, S., and J. Lumley. "Maternal Health after Childbirth: Results of an Australian Population-based Survey." *British Journal of Obstetrics and Gynaecology* 105 (1998): 156–61.

Brubaker, L. "Outcomes of Trial of Labor after Previous Cesarean Delivery." *American Journal of Obstetrics and Gynecology* 186, no. 5 (May 2002): 1105–1106.

———. "Postpartum Urinary Incontinence." [letter]. *British Medical Journal* 324 (May 25, 2002): 1227–28.

Cardozo, L., A. Hextall, J. Bailey, et al. "Colposuspension after Previous Failed Incontinence Surgery: A Prospective Observational Study." *British Journal of Obstetrics and Gynaecology* 106 (April 1999): 340–44.

Corcos, J., S. Beaulieu, J. Donovan, et al. "Symptom Quality of Life Assessment Committee of the First International Consultation on Incontinence: Quality of Life Assessment in Men and Women with Urinary Incontinence." [review] *Journal of Urology* 168, no. 3 (September 2002): 896–905.

Dahl, Gail J. *Pregnancy & Childbirth Tips.* Vancouver: Innovative Publishing, 1998.

Dainer, M., C. D. Hall, J. Choe, et al. "The Burch Procedure: A Comprehensive Review." *Obstetrics and Gynecological Survey* 54, no. 1 (January 1999): 49–60.

Day, M. H. "Posture and Childbirth." In *The Cambridge Encyclopedia of Human Evolution.* Edited by S. Jones et al. New York: Cambridge University Press, 1992.

Deindl, F. M., D. B. Vodusek, U. Hesse, et al. "Pelvic Floor Activity Patterns: Comparisons of Nulliparous Continent and Parous Urinary Stress Incontinent Women: A Kinesiological EMG Study." *British Journal of Urology* 73 (1994): 413–17.

Delancey, J. O. "Fascial and Muscular Abnormalities in Women with Urethral Hypermobility and Anterior Vaginal Wall Prolapse." *American Journal of Obstetrics and Gynecology* 187, no. 1 (July 2002): 93–98.

Dunn, S., I. Kowanko, J. Patterson, et al. "Systematic Review of the Effectiveness of Urinary Incontinence Products." [review]. *Journal of Wound, Ostomy, and Continence Nursing* 29, no. 3 (May 2002): 129–42.

Evrard, J. R., and E. M. Gold. "Cesarean Section and Maternal Mortality in Rhode Island." *Obstetrics and Gynecology* 50, no. 5 (November 1977): 594–97.

Fallouji, M. A. "Arabic Caesarean Section: Islamic History and Current Practice." *Scottish Medical Journal* 38, no.1 (February 1993): 30.

Fitzgerald, M. P., N. Butler, S. Shott, et al. "Bother Arising from Urinary Frequency in Women." *Neurology and Urodynamics* 21, no. 1 (2002): 36–40.

Forster, F. M. "Caesarean Section and Its Early Australian History." *Medical Journal of Australia* 4, no. 2 (July 1970): 33–38.

Frigoletto, F. D., K. J. Ryan, and M. Phillippe. "Maternal Mortality Rate Associated with Cesarean Section: An Appraisal." *American Journal of Obstetrics and Gynecology* 136 (1980): 969.

Frudinger, A., S. Halligan, and C. I. Bartram, et al. "Changes in Anal Anatomy Following Vaginal Delivery Revealed by Anal Endoscopy." *British Journal of Obstetrics and Gynaecology* 106 (March 1999): 233–37.

Futuyama, Douglas J. *Science on Trial: The Case for Evolution.* Sunderland, Mass.: Sinauer Associates, 1995.

Gjessing, H., B. Backe, and Y. Sahlin. "Third Degree Obstetric Tears: Outcome after Primary Repair." *Acta Obstetricia et Gynecologica Scandinavica* 77 (1998): 736–40.

Glazener, C. M. A. "Sexual Function after Childbirth: Women's Experiences, Persistent Morbidity and Lack of Professional Recognition." *British Journal of Obstetrics and Gynaecology* 104 (1997): 330–35.

Goffeng, A. R., B. Andersch, M. Andersson, et al. "Objective Methods Cannot Predict Anal Incontinence after Primary Repair of Extensive Anal Tears." *Acta Obstetricia et Gynecologica Scandinavica* 77, no. 4 (April 1998): 439–43.

Graham, W. J., V. Hundley, A. L. McCheyne, et al. "An Investigation of Women's Involvement in the Decision to Deliver by Caesarean Section." *British Journal of Obstetrics and Gynaecology* 106 (March 1999): 213–20.

Greene, J. C. *The Death of Adam: Evolution and Its Impact on Western Thought.* 1959. Reprint, Ames: Iowa State University Press, 1966.

Grill, W. M., M. D. Craggs, R. D. Foreman, et al. "Emerging Clinical Applications of Electrical Stimulation: Opportunities for Restoration of Function." [review] *Journal of Rehabilitation Research and Development* 38, no. 6 (November–December 2001): 641–53.

Grubb, J. M. "The First Successful Cesarean Section and the First Oophorectomy in the Americas." *West Virginia Medical Journal* 80, no. 10 (October 1984): 221–23.

Haadem, K., and S. Gudmundsson. "Can Women with Intrapartum Rupture of Anal Sphincter Still Suffer After-Effects Two Decades Later?" *Acta Obstetricia et Gynecologica Scandinavica* 76 (1997): 601–603.

Hagglund, D., H. Olsson, and J. Leppert. "Urinary Incontinence: An

Unexpected Large Problem among Young Females: Results from a Population-based Study." *Family Practice* 16, no. 5 (1999): 506–509.

Hayat, S. K., J. M. Thorp Jr., J. A. Kuller, et al. "Magnetic Resonance Imaging of the Pelvic Floor in the Postpartum Patient." *International Urogynecology Journal and Pelvic Floor Dysfunction* 7, no. 6 (1996): 321–24.

Hay-Smith, J., P. Herbison, and S. Morkved. "Physical Therapies for Prevention of Urinary and Faecal Incontinence in Adults." [review] *Cochrane Database of Systematic Reviews* 2 (2002): CDO033191.

Heit, M., K. Mudd, and P. Culligan. "Prevention of Childbirth Injuries to the Pelvic Floor." [review] *Current Women's Health Reports* 1, no. 1 (August 2001): 72–80.

Hellman, L. M. "Postmortem Cesarean Section." *American Journal of Obstetrics and Gynecology* 111, no. 8 (December 15, 1971): 1123.

Hemmer, H. "A New View of the Evolution of Man." *Current Anthropology* 10, nos. 2–3 (April–June 1969): 179–80.

Hogberg, U. "Maternal Deaths Related to Cesarean Section in Sweden, 1951–1980." *Acta Obstetricia et Gynecologica Scandinavica* 68, no. 4 (1989): 351–57.

Hojberg, K. E., J. D. Salvig, N. A. Winslow, et al. "Urinary Incontinence: Prevalence and Risk Factors at 16 Weeks of Gestation." *British Journal of Obstetrics and Gynaecology* 106 (August 1999): 842–50.

Houtzager, H. L. "Cesarean Section Till the End of the Sixteenth Century." *European Journal of Obstetrics, Gynecology, and Reproductive Biology* 13, no. 1 (February 1982): 57–58.

Hull, T. L., and J. W. Milsom. "Pelvic Floor Disorders." *Surgical Clinics of North America* 74, no. 6 (December 1994): 1399–1413.

James, T. "The Caesarean Operation." *South African Medical Journal* 44, no. 47 (November 28, 1970): 1359–63.

Janov, A. *The Feeling Child*. New York: Simon and Schuster, 1973.

Jolly, J., J. Walker, and K. Bhabra. "Subsequent Obstetric Performance Related to Primary Mode of Delivery." *British Journal of Obstetrics and Gynaecology* 106 (March 1999): 227–32.

Jongen, V. H. W. M., M. G. C. Halfwerk, and W. K. Brouwer. "Vaginal Delivery after Previous Caesarean Section for Failure of Second Stage of Labor." *British Journal of Obstetrics and Gynaecology* 105 (1998): 1079–81.

Jozwik, M. "The Physiological Basis of Pelvic Floor Exercises in the Treatment of Stress Urinary Incontinence." *British Journal of Obstetrics and Gynaecology* 105 (October 1998): 1046–51.

King, A. G. "America's First Cesarean Section." *Obstetrics and Gynecology* 37, no. 5 (May 1971): 797–802.

———. "The Legend of Jesse Bennet's 1794 Caesarian Section." *Bulletin of the History of Medicine* 50, no. 2 (summer 1976): 242–50.

King, J. K., and R. M. Freeman. "Is Antenatal Bladder Neck Mobility a Risk Factor for Postpartum Stress Incontinence?" *British Journal of Obstetrics and Gynaecology* 105 (December 1998): 1300–1307.

Kobashi, K. C. "Pelvic Prolapse." *Journal of Urology* 164, no. 6 (December 2002): 1879–90.

Kohli, N. and J. R. Miklos. "Use of Synthetic Mesh and Donor Grafts in Gynecologic Surgery." [review] *Current Women's Health Reports* 1, no. 1 (August 2001): 53–60.

Kohli, N., and P. L. Rosenblatt. "Neuromodulation Techniques for the Treatment of the Overactive Bladder." [review] *Clinical Obstetrics and Gynecology* 45, no. 1 (March 2002): 218–32.

Mallipeddi, P. K. "Anatomic and Functional Outcome of Vaginal Paravaginal Repair in the Correction of Anterior Vaginal Wall Prolapse." *International Urogynecology Journal and Pelvic Floor Dysfunction* 12, no. 2 (January 2001): 83–88.

Marshall, K., K. A. Thompson, and O. M. Walsh, et al. "Incidence of Urinary Incontinence and Constipation during Pregnancy and Postpartum: Survey of Current Findings at the Rotunda Lying-in Hospital." *British Journal of Obstetrics and Gynaecology* 105 (1998): 400–402.

McCandlish, R., U. Bowler, H. van Asten, et al. "A Randomised Controlled Trial of Care of the Perineum during Second Stage of Normal Labor." *British Journal of Obstetrics and Gynaecology* 105 (December 1998): 1262–72.

McCrone, J. *Going Inside: A Tour Round a Single Moment of Consciousness*. London: Faber and Faber, 1999.

Miklos, J. R., and N. Kohli. "Laparoscopic Paravaginal Repair Plus Burch Colposuspension: Review and Descriptive Technique." [review] *Urology* 56 (December 2000): 64–69.

Miklos, J. R., N. Kohli, and R. D. Moore. "Laparoscopic Management of Urinary Incontinence, Ureteric and Bladder Injuries."

[review] *Current Opinion in Obstetrics & Gynecology* 13, no. 4 (August 2001): 411–17.

Millar, W. J., C. Nair, and S. Wadhera. "Declining Cesarean Section Rates: A Continuing Trend?" *Health Reports* 8, no. 1 (1996): 17–24.

Miller, J. M. "First Successful Cesarean Section in the British Empire." [letter] *American Journal of Obstetrics and Gynecology* 166 (January 1992): 269.

Monga, A. "Fascia—Defects and Repair." *Current Opinion in Obstetrics and Gynecology* 8, no. 5 (October 1996): 366–71.

Moore, R. D., S. E. Speights, and J. R. Miklos. "Laparoscopic Burch Colposuspension for Recurrent Stress Urinary Incontinence." *Journal of the American Association of Gynecologic Laparoscopists* 8, no. 8 (August 2001): 389–92.

Morton, G. R. *Adam, Apes and Anthropology*. Dallas: DMD Publishing, 1997.

Mucrunski, M. "Average Charges for Uncomplicated Vaginal, Cesarean and VBAC Deliveries: Regional Variations, United States, 1996." *Statistics Bulletin Metropolitan Life Insurance Company* 79, no. 3 (July 1998): 17–28.

Naqvi, N. H. "James Barlow (1767–1839): Operator of the First Successful Caesarean Section in England." *British Journal of Obstetrics and Gynaecology* 92, no. 5 (May 1985): 468–72.

Nipe, G. M. "Jessee Bennett Decided to Operate on His Wife at Once." *Virginia Medical Quarterly* 106, no. 12 (December 1979): 884–85.

Norton, P. A. "Pelvic Floor Disorders: The Role of Fascia and Ligaments." *Clinical Obstetrics and Gynecology* 36, no. 4 (December 1993): 926–38.

Ostergard, D. R., and A. E. Bent. *Urogynecology and Urodynamics Theory and Practice*. 4th ed. Baltimore: Williams and Wilkins, 1996.

Paddison, K. "Complying with Pelvic Floor Exercises: A Literature Review." [review] *Nursing Standard* 16, no. 39 (June 12–18, 2002): 33–38.

Pemberton, J. H., M. Swash, and M. M. Henry, eds. *The Pelvic Floor: Its Functions and Disorders*. London: W. B. Saunders, 2002.

Peschers, V., G. Schaer, C. Anthuber, et al. "Changes in Vesical Neck Mobility Following Vaginal Delivery." *Obstetrics and Gynecology* 88, no. 6 (December 1996): 1001–1006.

Petitti, D. B. "Maternal Mortality and Morbidity in Cesarean Section." *Clinical Obstetrics and Gynecology* 28, no. 4 (December 1985): 763–69.

Richardson, A. C. "Female Pelvic Floor Support Defects." *International Urogynecology Journal of Pelvic Floor Dysfunction* 7, no. 5 (1996): 241.

———. "The Rectovaginal Septum Revisited: Its Relationship to Rectocele and Its Importance in Rectocele Repair." *Clinical Obstetrics and Gynecology* 36, no. 4 (December 1993): 976–83.

Rieger, N., A. Schloithe, G. Saccone, et al. "The Effect of a Normal Vaginal Delivery on Anal Function." *Obstetrical & Gynecological Survey* 53, no. 6 (June 1998): 345–46.

Rieger, N., and D. Wattchow. "The Effect of Vaginal Delivery on Anal Function." *Australian and New Zealand Journal of Surgery* 69 (1999): 172–77.

Rosenthal, A. N., and S. Paterson-Brown. "Is There an Incremental Rise in the Risk of Obstetric Intervention with Increasing Maternal Age?" *British Journal of Obstetrics and Gynaecology* 105 (October 1998): 1064–69.

Rubin, G. L., H. B. Peterson, R. W. Rochat, et al. "Maternal Death after Cesarean Section in Georgia." *American Journal of Obstetrics and Gynecology* 139, no. 6 (March 15, 1981): 681–85.

Ruff, C. B. "Climate and Body Shape in Hominid Evolution." *Journal of Human Evolution* 21 (1991): 81–105.

Sachs, B. P., J. Yeh, D. Acker, et al. "Cesarean Section-Related Maternal Mortality in Massachusetts, 1954–1985." *Obstetrics and Gynecology* 71 (March 1998): 385–88.

Schuitemaker, N., J. van Roosmalen, G. Dekker, et al. "Maternal Mortality after Cesarean Section in The Netherlands." *Acta Obstetricia et Gynecologica Scandinavica* 76, no. 4 (April 1997): 332–34.

Shreeve, James R. *The Neandertal Enigma*. London: Penguin Books, 1995.

Shute, W. B. "Save Those Marriages with Mediolateral Episiotomies." *Medical Post* 35, no. 3 (January 19, 1999): 15.

Simeonova, Z., I. Milson, A. Kullenorff, et al. "The Prevalence of Urinary Incontinence and Its Influence on the Quality of Life in Women from an Urban Swedish Population." *Acta Obstetricia et Gynecologica Scandinavica* 78 (1999): 546–51.

Snooks, S. J., M. Swash, M. Setchell, et al. "Injury to Innervation of

Pelvic Floor Sphincter Musculature in Childbirth." *Lancet* 2, no. 8402 (September 8, 1984): 546–50.

Speights, S. E., R. D. Moore, and J. R. Miklos. "Frequency of Lower Urinary Tract Injury at Laparoscopic Burch and Paravaginal Repair." *Journal of the American Association of Gynecologic Laparoscopists* 7, no. 4 (November 2000): 515–18.

Steer, P. "Caesarean Section: An Evolving Procedure?" *British Journal of Obstetrics and Gynaecology* 105 (October 1998): 1052–55.

———. "Fetal Growth." *British Journal of Obstetrics and Gynaecology* 105 (November 1998): 1133–35.

Sultan, A. H., M. A. Kamm, and C. N. Hudson. "Pudendal Nerve Damage during Labor: Prospective Study Before and After Childbirth." *British Journal of Obstetrics and Gynaecology* 101 (January 1994): 22–28.

Sultan, A. H., M. A. Kamm, C. N. Hudson, et al. "Third-Degree Obstetric Anal Sphincter Tears: Risk Factors and Outcome of Primary Repair." *British Medical Journal* 308, no. 6933 (April 2, 1994): 887–91.

Thompson, P. K., R. J. Mooney, A. Plummer, et al. "Paravaginal Plus? A Better Incontinence Operation?" *Journal of Pelvic Surgery* 4 (1998): 157–62.

Thorp, J. M., P. A. Norton, L. L. Wall, et al. "Urinary Incontinence in Pregnancy and the Puerperium: A Prospective Study." *American Journal of Obstetrics and Gynecology* 181, no. 2 (year): 266–73.

Toglia, M. R., and J. O. L. DeLancey. "Anal Incontinence and the Obstetrician-Gynecologist." *Obstetrics and Gynecology* 84 (October 1994): 731–40.

Trevathan, Wenda R. *Human Birth: An Evolutionary Perspective*. New York: Aldine de Gruyter, 1987.

Ulmsten, U., and P. Petros. "Intravaginal Slingplasty (IVS): An Ambulatory Surgical Procedure for Treatment of Female Urinary Incontinence." *Scandinavian Journal of Urology and Nephrology* 29 (March 1995): 75–82.

Ulmsten, U., P. Johnson, and M. Rezapour. "A Three-Year Followup of Tension Free Vaginal Tape for Surgical Treatment of Female Stress Urinary Incontinence." *British Journal of Obstetrics and Gynaecology* 106 (April 1999): 345–50.

Upadhyay, N., R. Buist, and M. Selinger. "Caesarian Section: An Evolving Procedure?" [letter] *British Journal of Obstetrics and Gynaecology* 106 (March 1999): 286–87.

Visco, A. G., and C. Figuers. "Nonsurgical Management of Pelvic Floor Dysfunction." *Obstetrics and Gynecology Clinics of North America* 25 (1998): 849–65.

Walker, A., and P. Shipman. *The Wisdom of the Bones*. New York: Alfred A. Knopf, 1996.

Walker, M. C., P. R. Garner, and E. J. Kelly. "Thrombosis in Pregnancy: A Review." *Journal of the Society of Obstetricians and Gynaecologists of Canada* 20, no. 10 (September 1998): 943–52.

Wall, L. L. "The Muscles of the Pelvic Floor." *Clinical Obstetrics and Gynecology* 36, no. 4 (December 1993): 910–25.

Wallin, G. and O. Fall. "Modified Joel-Cohen Technique for Caesarean Delivery." *British Journal of Obstetrics and Gynaecology* 106 (March 1999): 221–26.

Weidner, A. C. "Article Name." *American Journal of Obstetrics and Gynecology* 183, no. 6 (December 2000): 1390–1401.

Wilson, D. J., and M. J. Douglas. "Spinal Anaesthesia for Caesarian Section." *Journal of the Society of Obstetricians and Gynaecologists of Canada* 20, no. 8 (July 1998): 754–61.

Zetterstrom, J. P., A. Lopez, B. Anzen, et al. "Anal Incontinence after Vaginal Delivery: Prospective Study in Primiparous Women." *British Journal of Obstetrics and Gynaecology* 106 (April 1999): 324–30.

Zivkovic, F., and K. Tamussino. "Effects of Vaginal Surgery on the Lower Urinary Tract." *Current Opinion in Obstetrics & Gynecology* 9 (1997): 329–31.

About the Authors

Dr. Magnus Murphy resides in Calgary, Canada, with his wife and two daughters. He is a specialist in treating patients with pelvic floor disorders, and is one of the first Canadian gynecologists to introduce the new TVT procedure for urinary stress incontinence into his practice. He is currently a clinical assistant professor within the Department of Obstetrics and Gynecology in Calgary, and is in private practice, having spent seven years as a specialist obstetrician and gynecologist in British Columbia. Other previous positions include: Chairman, Department of Obstetrics, Cranbrook Regional Hospital; and Acting Chief of Staff, Prince Rupert Regional Hospital.

He attended medical school at the University of Stellenbosch in South Africa. Following his internship at Windhoek State Hospital in Namibia, Africa, he served as a lieutenant and medical officer for the South African Defense Force Medical Service. During that time he provided healthcare to Third-World regions where women with severe pelvic floor disorders literally become sexual and social outcasts isolated from their tribes and live in desperation and shame.

In 1995, Dr. Murphy relocated to Canada where he obtained a Fellowship from the Royal College of Surgeons of Canada and the Society of Obstetricians and Gynecologists of Canada (SOGC). He is a frequent delegate, speaker, and panelist at SOCG conferences and Women's Health conferences.

Carol L. Wasson is a veteran freelance nonfiction writer and an internationally published industry trade press author. Additionally, as a marketing and public relations consultant, she is the owner of JCL Marketing and Communications, Inc., a company that provides communications programs to corporate clients. Wasson resides with her husband, daughter, and many beloved animals in the rural countryside of Decatur, Indiana.

Index